COMBO
CISING

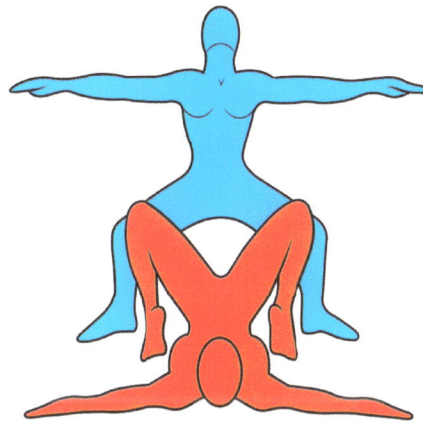

The Science of Toning The Body and Relationship
Through Muscle Toning Exercises and
Love Making Techniques.

Written by
KEITH RIDDICK

Design & Illustration by
JOSHUA ROCH

Additional Illustration by
ALWING LOPEZ-LEWIS

To, God, Family, and Friends

SPECIAL THANKS

First and foremost I want to thank GOD for the many blessing bestowed upon me. I would like to thank him for giving me the wisdom, insight, and relentless spirit to bring this dream to fruition.

Secondly I would like to thank my beautiful and patient wife, Sheila for her support during this project and enduring many hours of me rambling on about this book. I also need to thank my children Bria, Askia, and Mya. I have sacrificed many opportunities to spend time with them for the sake of this book. My hope is that they understand why daddy did what he did.

I want to thank my dear friend James Jackson, Ph.D. for his contribution and support at the conception of this project. It was the look in his eyes when I first mentioned it to him that told me I was onto something.

In addition, I would like to thank Joshua Roche and Alwing Lewis, two brilliant and talented illustrators with whom I hope to work with **on** future projects.

There are two dear people to whom I owe a great amount of thanks for their moral and economic support. To my sister, Patsy Harris who has been like a mother figure to me since I was a child, I give thanks. You hold the family down since the passing of our mother, becoming the beacon, leading our family through dark times.

Finally, I would like to thank Mike Saraceno. This man has proven to be more than just a friend he is my brother. He saw my vision and never lost faith in it. So to Mike and those loved ones not here to witness the publication of this book, I give thanks.

FORWARD

In recent decades, researchers and psychologist have come to understand the importance of physical exercise in healthy adult life style. It's not surprising that a good diet, a sensible exercise program, and a significant amount of rest, have been found to be the fountain of youth. Combocising brings together all these factors in a unique and innovative way.

In recent reports by the government, it's been stated that over 50% of all marriages end in divorce or separation. One of the leading causes for this phenomenon is a lack of intimate interaction between couples. Intimate interaction can be defined in several different ways; one being quality time, which has become the newest "buzzword".

Combocising is an exceptional prospect for increasing the amounts of intimate interaction, or quality time between couples. Combocising combines physical exercise and quality time, for couples seeking to increase their healthy adult life-style, while providing a new way of getting to know each other.

Combocising blends together the qualities of healthy intimate interaction between couples. These qualities are physical closeness, helpful behavior, expression of a caring nature and personal self-disclosure. By combining these qualities within a framework of a high quality work out, Combocising provides couples with an appropriate structure to increase their overall physical fitness while working on their relationships.

James D. Jackson Phd.
Kutztown University
Kutztown Pennsylvania

TABLE OF CONTENTS

INTRODUCTION 6

CHAPTER ONE
THE OBSESSION 9

CHAPTER TWO
EXERCISE AND FITNESS 19

CHAPTER THREE
WARM-UP AND FOREPLAY 22

CHAPTER FOUR
EXERCISE AND SEX 28

CHAPTER FIVE
COOL DOWN AND POST-PLAY 64

TIPS 65

CHAPTER SIX
MASSAGE 66

CHAPTER SEVEN
NUTRITION AND DIETING 72

ADDITIONAL WEIGHT LOSS AND MAINTENANCE TIPS 80

CHAPTER EIGHT
EXERCISE AND RELATIONSHIPS 81

AUTHOR'S NOTES 83

SAMPLE WORKOUTS 84

TRAINING LOG 87

REFERENCE PAGE 95

INTRODUCTION

One Saturday, approximately nine and a half years ago, I sat in my living room watching television when an infomercial came on promoting a product called the Bun and Body Sculptor. In the beginning, this apparatus seemed no different from the many other products that were already flooding the market, but as the commercial went on, my interest began to peak for several reasons:

- The beauty of the model demonstrating the exercises.

- The body parts the cameraperson focused on.

- The sexual overtones during the commercial.

- The needs and desires of the target market group (women).

There were two things that I saw and heard during this infomercial that changed my views on exercising forever. They were: the needs and desires of women and the desires and needs of men.

The needs and desires of most women were pretty simple—they wanted to work out three times a week, thirty minutes a day, in the comfort of their own homes. The main reasons given by these women for wanting to work out in their homes were: convenience and avoiding remarks and uninvited stares by men when performing certain exercises in compromising positions.

For example, one such exercise is the bent leg lift. This particular exercise requires the woman to be positioned on the floor, resting on her knees and elbows (doggy style), with a resistance bar across the back of her thigh. During this exercise, she raises her leg in the extended direction (back), working the hamstring and gluteus maximus muscles.

As you can imagine, this exposes her buttocks to all male and female onlookers, which can be a terrifying experience to a person who is very self-conscious. Another such position was the pelvic thrust, where the woman lies in a supine (missionary) position, with her legs approximately shoulder-width apart, bent at a 45-degree angle, and with a resistance bar placed across her pelvic region. During this exercise, she raises her buttocks off the mat, expelling the air as she pulls the abdominal muscles in toward the lower back and curls the pelvis up toward the navel.

This exercise in particular caught my attention because this was a move that had been performed on me by past lovers and my wife while being intimate. As I reflected on those moments, I pondered the thought, "What if the man became the resistance bar by applying his body weight and vice versa for the woman?" The idea intrigued me, and I began to brainstorm putting exercises to sexual positions.

The statements made and the exercises performed during the infomercial happened to correspond to an article I found in a 1998 *Reader's Digest* magazine entitled, "Surprising Health Benefi ts of Sex." "Sexual activity is a form of physical exercise," says Dr. Mchael Cirigliano, assistant professor of medicine at the University of Pennsylvania School of Medicine. The article suggested that having modest sex three times a week annually could burn 7,500 calories per year, which is the equivalent of jogging 75 miles. If performed more vigorously, you can burn up to ten thousand calories per year, or the equivalent of one hundred miles.

Sex has such medicinal benefits as increased HDL levels (cholesterol) and increased testosterone. "Regular lovemaking can also increase levels of estrogen, which protects the heart and keeps **vaginal tissues supple," says clinical psychologist Karen Donahey, director of the Sex and Marital Therapy Program at Northwestern University Medical School. Other benefi ts include relief from stress, which is known to weaken the immune system, causing people to become more susceptible to illness. Another benefi t is the squeezing of excess fl uids from the prostate that is not adequately drained, a condition common among men in their late forties. This is done by the muscle contractions during orgasm.**

With all this information in hand, I thought to myself, "What if exercises were performed while couples were intimate? Could this be the carrot that dangles so temptingly in front of the mule, enticing him to perform? (Excuse the metaphorical pun.)

Could it also be the incentive to encourage some of the 60 percent of Americans who do not get the daily required amount of exercise and the 25 percent who are totally sedentary to find some interest in staying fit and healthy?"

My other thought was that it might also aid the one million couples that get legally divorced every year and those unmarried individuals who go through headaches and heartbreaks but are otherwise unaccounted for.

So after nearly ten years of research, education, and personal growth, it has culminated into *COMBOCISING: The Science of Toning the Body and Relationship Through Muscle Toning Exercises and Lovemaking Techniques.*

I do not pretend to think that Combocising is a cure all for the many issues that plague couples today. But I do believe that if couples who have invested great amounts of time and emotion in their relationships can reestablish their commitment and find common ground on which they can grow, they will have a much better and healthier chance of surviving in our modern-day society.

CHAPTER ONE
THE OBSESSION

At any given time across this country, countless millions from all walks of life are engaging in one or two of American society's most popular activities. These are fitness and sex. These two subjects command great attention in our culture. As a matter of fact, we are obsessed with them.

If there is any doubt about the validity of this statement, take a moment and check out the magazine rack at the corner store or the checkout line of your favorite grocer: *THE SEX ISSUE! A 25 PAGE SPECIAL ON AMERICA'S FAVORITE PASTIME, Burn Fat and Get Fit, The 7 Best Sex Tips You've Ever Heard* ... etc. There is article after article on the topics of fitness and sex. Sex and fitness dominate the covers of most contemporary magazines and even some that our parents may have subscribed to, such as *Reader's Digest*.

Fit figures and ultraslim models **grace** the covers of magazines, big screens, walkways, and televisions, setting the standard by which all others are to be measured. We have become a nation of idolaters (idol worshipers). These images represent the way mass media thinks we should look and many have bought into the philosophy. It is thought that if you look sexy, you are fit, and if you look fit, you are sexy.

The sex industry, which consists of everything from movies, adult toys, magazines, and lingerie, is a multibillion-dollar-a-year industry. The fitness industry is no less profitable, at nearly two hundred billion dollars a year, with tremendous growth potential. There are several factors that will contribute to this growth:

- The recent Surgeon General's report estimates 60 percent of America does not receive the daily recommended amount of exercise, and 25 percent are totally sedentary.
- The alarming number of cases of obesity in this country.
- We have one of the worst diets in the industrialized world, consisting mostly of meats and starches.
- Exercise and other health alternatives are starting to gain more and more acceptance in our society.

One other factor—if not the most important of them all—is our obsession (VANITY) with our external appearance. Hundreds of millions, even billions, are spent annually on everything from cosmetic surgery and pills to supplements and home training equipment. This is all done in an attempt to fulfill our narcissistic desire to be appealing and accepted by others. However, this mentality comes with great consequences to bear.

For instance, we have young girls in this country that believe that they must do one of two things in order for them to make it in our society. The first is to starve themselves into an anorectic or bulimic state so they may appear statuesque. The other is to get a pair of implanted breasts, believing this will get them the attention and status they need and desire.

Young men are injecting themselves with steroids and other growth-enhancing hormones, not realizing the internal damage that is occurring to the heart, kidneys, and liver. They are trying to become the Barbie dolls and action figures they once played with as children.

Our perception of health and fitness has been distorted and grossly misrepresented, partly out of ignorance, but mostly in the name of capitalism. In our modern-day society, everyone wants to look and feel sexy, from preteen girls to golden-girl grannies. These two age groups and everyone in between frolic around scantly clad, trying to catch someone's eye because they know that sex sells.

We all like some amount of attention, and looking and feeling sexy does something for a person's self-confidence. Perhaps this is the reason it has become a social tool, a means of fitting in and reaching one's end. But there are many people out there who are sexually unfulfilled. They are in continual search for tips and outlandish ideas on how to please their mate and be pleased themselves.

I once read in a magazine that 60 percent of women have never experienced an orgasm. Most of the blame seems to be placed on the man's failure to be more attentive to the woman's needs. Women say that men don't take the time to explore the woman's body, seeking her erogenous zones. Then when these points are located, they don't spend the necessary time to bring them to fulfillment.

In a book entitled *Sexual Fitness*, by Hank C. K. Wuh, MD and Meikei Fox, the authors suggest that all women have the ability to have an orgasm, and it takes a minimum of fifteen minutes to bring a woman to sexual orgasm. To a lot of men, that is a long time and seems like a lot of work, especially when they are accustomed to having their desires met and not having to meet the desires of another.

In one such case, a coworker told me about a situation he was having in his newly formed relationship. He had met a woman after recently being divorced from his wife of nineteen years. In the beginning, everything seemed great (as it always does), but within a month or two, he felt as though he might want to see other people. His dilemma was that he had feelings for this woman, but he felt that they might be sexually incompatible. His reasoning for this was that she took a long time to reach her orgasm, and he was not accustomed to working that hard. He was used to women climaxing upon his touch (figuratively speaking), so when this did not happen with this woman, I believe his ego was somewhat shaken.

He did however express a willingness to try new things but did not know how to approach her about it without hurting her feelings. I suggested to him that he run a tub of hot water filled with bubbles and add some candles and soft music to create a relaxing atmosphere.

By doing this, it took them out of the places they generally had discussions and put them in a warm and inviting environment where they could open up to one another. I told him to bring it up in a way that was nonthreatening to her, by maybe mentioning that a coworker was writing a workout manual for couples. If she showed an interest in it, then he would know she was open for new things as well. If she did not, then maybe he would have to pursue another course of action.

I left the job site that day and haven't seen this person since, but the moral of this story is that everyone responds to touch differently! What worked with previous lovers may not work for the next, so take the time and explore the person's body and mind.

It is important for people to understand that the skin (sometimes refereed to as the cutaneous membrane) of the human body is the largest organ of the human body. It has millions of sensory receptors collecting information called sensory input. The sensory input is converted into electrical signals called nerve impulses, which are transmitted to the brain.

At this point, the signals are brought together to create sensations, thoughts, or to add to memory. This is why it is said that the brain is the greatest sexual organ—because it is the stimuli (sensory input) during sexual encounters that bring the mind to a climactic or orgasmic state. The resulting effect is the release of the nectar, or love juices.

Figure 1-1 on page 13 offers a combonation where one partner stretches to loosen the upper torso, shoulders, and arms while the other performs squats. This combonation allows the person performing the squats to explore their partner's body using the senses of touch, smell, taste, and, of course, sight. The fifth sense, hearing, will be used if you are attentive enough to bring them to an excited state and observant enough to listen for a change in their breathing pattern, which is an indication of arousal.

COMBONATION #1
STRETCHES AND SQUATS

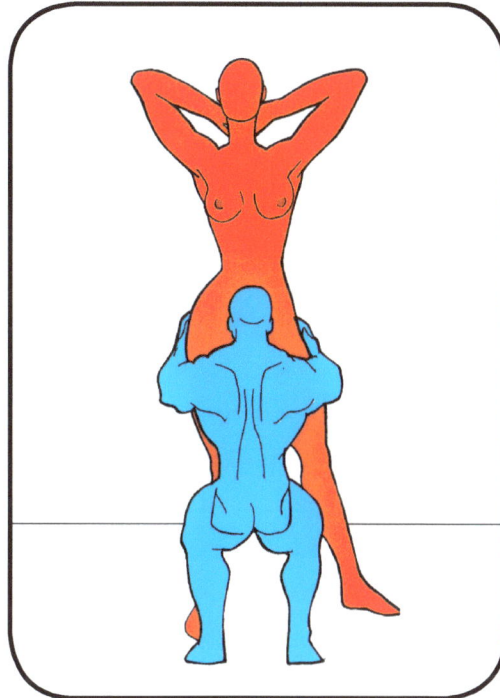

Figure 1-1

Muscles worked:

Man: Quadriceps femoris group and gluteus maximus .

Woman: Latissimus dorsi, triceps brachii

Slightly off center, and with their feet shoulder-width apart, both the man and woman stand facing one another, with the man placing his hands on the woman's waistline. This offers stability and provides an opportunity for the man or woman to use his/her hands to help explore the other's erogenous zones.

The man slowly lowers himself to the squat position, kissing, licking, and smelling the woman on the way down and doing the same to the up position. The woman will perform triceps and latissimus dorsi stretches by dropping one hand behind her head, using the opposite hand to grab the elbow, then performing lateral flexion (bending side to side). Back extensions can also be performed during this exercise. Perform 3 sets of squats for 10–12 reps then switch.

KEITH RIDDICK | 13

It is time to put things into proper perspective when addressing what is perceived as the shortcomings of the man. Again, pardon the pun. It is imperative that both men and women understand the psychological and physiological similarities and differences between orgasm and ejaculation.

The act of orgasm, which is more commonly associated with the pleasures of a woman than that of a man, is a peak experience that follows intense arousal.

The authors of the book *The Multi-Orgasmic Woman*—Mantak Chia and Rachel Carlton Abrams, MD, define orgasm for the woman as the pleasurable contraction of the pelvic floor, or pubococcygeus (PC) muscle, and the smooth muscle of the vagina and uterus.

But recent studies show that men are not only capable of having an orgasm, but multiple orgasms. Orgasm for the man occurs just prior to ejaculation and is described as a wave of sexual euphoria, but he must be attuned to his body to know when this occurs. A better understanding of this can been found in the book *The Multi–Orgasmic Man*, by Mantak Chia. In this book, the author explains how men can learn how to recognize this orgasmic state and increase their sexual pleasure.

Now, the act of ejaculation for most healthy men is the end result of a process culminating in the production of sperm cells for the purpose of procreation. During this process, several organs contribute to the production and release of millions of sperm cells, which is very taxing on the body. This helps to explain why men often become fatigued after ejaculation.

Often, the man can maintain an erection after ejaculation for a short period of time or even continue on, depending on his age and physical and sexual fitness. Failure to get or maintain an erection during sex can also be a sign of coronary or vascular disease. If this occurs, you should see your doctor.

In most cases, however, the blood that was diverted from the different organs of the body to engorge the penis returns to its normal path of flow once the stimulus is removed.

This begins the *Refractory Period*, which is defined as the period of time during which a point on the cell membrane is "recovering" from depolarization. While the membrane is permeable to sodium ions, it cannot respond to a second stimulus, no matter how strong the stimulus.

The refractory period, as it relates to the male erection, is the time between the man's first erection and his ability to gain another. This recovery period in healthy men can vary from as little as five minutes to fifteen minutes. During this period, you can gain significant points and buy time by holding each other or just having meaningful conversation. After the refractory period has ended, you and your partner can resume the lovemaking session, if so desired.

But how long is a lovemaking, sex-having, or fucking session (excuse my French) supposed to last? Fifteen, thirty, sixty minutes—longer, maybe? I do not wish to offend anyone by using what is perceived to be vulgar language, but *fuck* is not a word, it is an acronym, which stands for Fornication Under Consent of the King. It is actually old English, not French. As part of my research, I observed the mating habits of several animal and insect species, most of which was conducted by watching the Learning and Discovery channels.

However, I was able to watch my dogs as well as earthworms and other insect groups mate firsthand and discovered that procreation generally lasted no more than ten to fifteen minutes on average.

This seemed pretty consistent throughout the animal and insect kingdoms. (Keep in mind that they did this for procreation and not recreation.) I continued on with my study on sexual behavior, shifting my focus to the practices and habits of humans. As a union electrician and an instructor at one of the nation's most recognized training facilities, I was afforded a large body of specimens to examine and obtain information from. Over the years, I listened to a lot of men complain about their problems with their wives and girlfriends. Among the many complaints these men had, sex, or the lack thereof, seemed to be the most common.

On the flip side, the women did not complain so much about the lack of sex as much as they did about the lack of affection and the man's inability to stimulate her mentally as well as physically.

Could it be that these women had become comfortable in their roles as wives and mothers and no longer felt it necessary to please their husbands after several years of marriage, as they had done during their courtship? Or did these men become insensitive to the wants and needs of their wives, causing the women to lose interest in them sexually?

I do not wish to point fingers or place blame on anyone because it takes a minimum of two people to hold intelligent conversation. But what I will say is this: both men and women should want to be more attentive to the other's needs because there are great fruits to be harvested from your labor if you are.

Many years ago, I theorized that it behooves a man to please a woman first, and in return he shall receive great pleasure. For instance, when women have orgasms, several things occur that will greatly enhance the experience for the man:

- The woman reaches that point of ecstasy that has many times eluded her and many others, so she will gladly reward your efforts.
- The vaginal cavity is thoroughly lubricated and allows for ease of penetration by the man.
- The pelvis tilts back, allowing for greater depth of penetration.
- Causing a woman to have multiple orgasms expends a great deal of energy, so much so that in most cases, the woman herself will fall asleep beside you or in your arms.

Figure 1-2 on page 18 illustrates a combonation that I am particularly fond of because of its versatility. Not only does it allow both individuals to work their abs and the woman to administer massage, you can also perform a technique I call wrestling.

The object of this exercise is to bring the woman to a multiple orgasmic state as the man attempts to hold her stationary. This exercise burns a tremendous amount of calories (calories are the unit for energy) and requires a certain level of endurance and strength. It also brings about an indescribable amount of pleasure.

I was once told that lovemaking is an art form. From that point on, I viewed it as such and took it upon myself to learn as much as I possibly could about the opposite sex. Sometimes it required me to read books and magazines or watch a television program or take the time to explore the woman's body myself. I enjoyed the latter the most, and I think that that course of action was the most appreciated.

I also asked dozens of women what was more important to them—the size of the man's penis or his ability to bring them to fulfillment? The overwhelming response was bringing them to fulfillment.

Yes, size does matter, in some cases, but size is not everything. So put aside all the myths and clichés and stop concerning yourself with things you have no control over and take control of the things you do.

COMBONATION #2
BRIDGES, ROLL UPS, AND MASSAGE

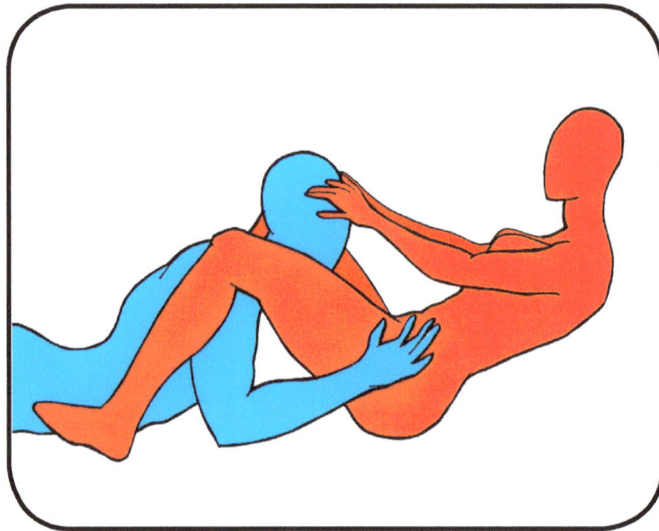

Figure 1-2

Muscles worked:

Man: Middle and upper rectus abdominis and transversus abdominis

Woman: Massage: Cranial and facial muscles

The woman lies in the supine position, with her legs apart, bent at a 45-degree angle. The man places himself down between her legs, lying in a prone position, resting on his elbows.

As the woman rises up to do partial sit-ups, the man also rises up on his toes and forearms doing the bridge, which exercises the abdominal muscles and torsal stabilizers by drawing the abdominal muscles up.

In this position, the man can kiss and lick her inner thighs and also orally massage the woman's clitoris. The woman can also administer massage to the face and head area of the man between sets. Woman: Do this for 10–12 reps for 3 sets. Man: hold each bridge for 10–15 sec. 5–10 reps.

CHAPTER TWO
EXERCISE AND FITNESS

Exercise is defined as activity for the purpose of training or developing the body or mind for the sake of health. *Fitness*, or *Physical Fitness*, on the other hand, is not so easily defined because it involves four separate components: 1) aerobic fitness; 2) muscle and joint flexibility; 3) muscle strength and endurance; and 4) body composition.

The majority of our nation's population is miseducated about what optimal fitness truly is. From my experience as a member of several large gym facilities and as a personal trainer in the field for the past six years, most people achieve maybe two of the components, or at best three.

The main focus of most individuals that start a fitness or weight-training program is not that of health but rather an issue of appearance. I must acknowledge those who do begin a program out of a concern for health, but even the majority of this group generally does so when health complications necessitate it.

With all the advancements in the fitness and weight training industry and a concerted effort to promote better health through fitness, recent reports indicate that less than 25 percent of the population is physically active.

Our society is besieged by health concerns, even though we are obsessed with fitness and dieting. This is understandable when you begin to understand that the term *diet* or *dieting* has been bastardized by corporate America.

Listen to me very closely: everything you eat is a part of your diet. I'll say this again: everything you eat is a part of your diet. Therefore, a person cannot go on a diet if they are already on a diet. Do you understand? Let me put it another way. You can only go on a diet if you have already stopped eating, and therein lies the problem. We are gluttons, eating more than we need to just because we can, and now we are faced with the issue of obesity.

Obesity can be summed up this way—32 percent body fat or higher for women and 25 percent body fat or higher for men. This condition is one of the leading causes of such health risks as hypertension, hyperlipidemia, osteoarthritis, and coronary artery disease.

According to ACE's (American Council on Exercise) Lifestyle and Weight Management Consultant manual, the percentage of overweight individuals in this country increased from 25 percent to 33 percent between 1976 and 1991. It is now 2006, and I'm sure those percentages are much higher today because of what we consume and the way we consume it.

The manual goes on to say that to successfully lose weight, it requires a multifaceted approach incorporating: sound nutrition, safe and effective physical activity, appropriate lifestyle changes, and psychological and emotional support. The perpetual search is on for the product or program that can arrest the attention and imagination of the American people.

The Lifestyle and Weight Management Consultant certification is sure to be of great benefit to the fitness professionals in helping those who are earnest about health and fitness. But what of the 75 percent or more who need coaxing?

What will it take to reach this group?

A variety of weight training and aerobic programs saturate the market, but one program is just a variation of another. Most are nothing more than fly-by-night gimmicks preying on people's weak emotional and psychological states, bilking consumers out of billions of dollars each year.

The program or product must offer variety because variety is important when participating in a fitness or aerobic program. One that lacks variety will quickly grow boring and dissatisfying and ultimately cause people to lose interest. That is why cross training is recommended.

A few of the latest exercise crazes are the stability ball, Pilates, and Tae Bo. All are good in their own right, but they are limited in the benefits they offer and the appeal to capture the masses.

Combocising is a program that not only offers a variety of exercises but a variety of benefits from those exercises that are not normally associated with the products currently on the market. Some examples of these are:

- Quality time with your significant other
- Spontaneity
- Stronger lines of communication
- Stronger commitment to each other's health and welfare

Please take note that the benefits listed are not physical ones that can easily be quantified. No! They are the intangibles that must be looked at over time and examined individually to help measure the success of your gains. This is where Combocising separates itself from other products on the market.

Where most products address the needs and desires of the individual, Combocising addresses the needs and desires of the individuals in relationships. This is achieved by making health the central focus and using exercise, massage, and intimacy as the vehicles to stimulate the mind and maintain the person's interest.

Combocising targets all the major muscle groups and many of the concerns of women and men, as previously mentioned.

We will now address each stage of the workout program (warm-up, exercise, and cooldown) and how it correlates to the act of intimacy (foreplay, sex, and post play).

CHAPTER THREE
WARM-UP AND FOREPLAY

Warm-up, in relation to physical activity, is defined as graduated low levels of aerobic exercise that maximize the safety and the economy of movement. The warm-up period gradually increases the heart rate, blood pressure, oxygen consumption, dilation of the blood vessels, elasticity of the active muscles, and the heat produced by the active muscle group.

The warm-up period is broken down into two distinct components: 1) Graduated aerobic activity such as walking or slow-tempo rhythmic calisthenic movements and 2) Flexibility exercise specific to the biomechanical nature of the primary conditioning activity (e.g., calf, quadriceps, and Achilles stretching before basketball or running). With regard to Combocising, slow rhythmic dancing will be combined with calisthenics.

Warm muscles are easier to stretch than cold muscles. An example of this can be demonstrated by bending a partially thawed piece of meat as compared to a fully thawed piece. Five to ten minutes of low-level aerobic activity using the targeted muscle groups followed by stretching of the same muscle group should precede the activity. Failure to do so may cause serious muscle, joint, and ligament damage.

Now, let us define foreplay and understand the correlation between it and the warm-up period. **Foreplay** is defined as mutual sexual stimulation preceding sexual intercourse. This stimulation can be in many forms and applied in a variety of ways, depending on the imagination of the parties involved.

As previously mentioned in chapter 1, the skin is the largest organ of the human body. It has millions of sensory receptors collecting information called sensory input. The sensory input is converted into electrical signals called nerve impulses, which are transmitted to the brain.

At this point, the signals are brought together to create sensations, thoughts, or to add to memory. This is why it is said that the brain is the greatest sexual organ—because it is the stimuli (sensory input) during sexual encounters that bring the mind to a climactic or orgasmic state. The resulting effect is the release of the nectar, or love juices.

This may sound redundant, but it bears repeating for two reasons: 1) People need to understand that the entire body is a sensory receptor, not just the clitoris, and 2) The warm-up period and foreplay both perform the same function in preparing the body for physical activity.

Since the warm-up period calls for graduated aerobic activity and flexibility exercises specific to the biomechanical nature of the primary conditioning activity, I had to think of what those activities would be in relation to Combocising. The choices were simple—dancing would be the graduated aerobic activity and assisted stretching would be the flexibility component.

Dancing has always been viewed as a sensual act of seduction, and in the last forty or so years has had an increased use in aerobic exercise. The aerobic aspect of dancing is nothing new, however. This art form dates back to many ancient cultures, where dance was a part of every ceremony and daily activity. Dancing will prepare the body by gradually increasing the heart rate, blood pressure, oxygen consumption, dilation of the blood vessels, elasticity of the active muscles, and the heat produced by the active muscle group. The slow and rhythmic movements of the pelvis will also send blood rushing to engorge the penis and clitoris while the assisted stretching will aid in muscle relaxation and prolonged foreplay.

Figures 3-1 through 3-4 on pages 24 through 27 demonstrate several assisted stretching techniques and foreplay ideas. Do not bounce (ballistic stretching) while stretching. This technique has a higher risk of injury and will only have short-term results. Whether you are assisted or alone, slowly and gradually go into each stretch and hold it for 10 seconds (static stretching). This will provide a longer-lasting and safer stretch.

Note: figure 3-1 is the same as the example figure 1-1 on page 13.

COMBONATION #1
STRETCHES AND SQUATS

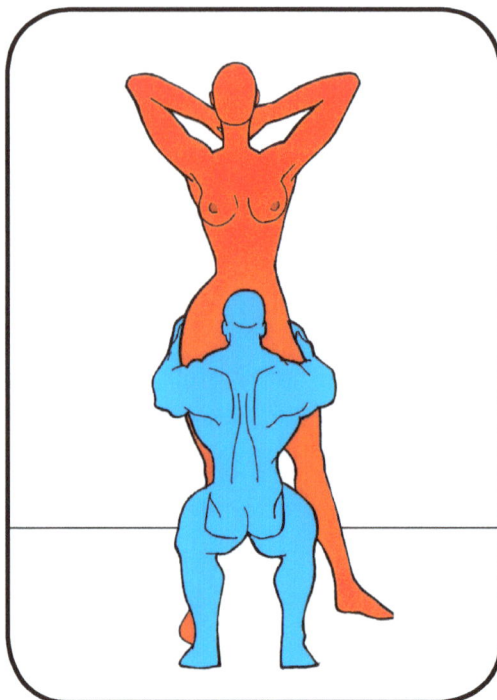

Figure 3-1

Muscles worked:

Man: Quadriceps femoris group and gluteus maximus

Woman: Latissimus dorsi, triceps brachii

Slightly off center, and their feet shoulder-width apart, both the man and woman stand facing one another, with the man placing his hands on the woman's waistline. This offers stability and provides an opportunity for the man or woman to use his/her hands to help explore the other's erogenous zones.

The man slowly lowers himself to the squat position, kissing, licking, and smelling the woman on the way down and doing the same to the up position. The woman will perform tricep and latissimus dorsi stretches, by dropping one hand behind her head, using the opposite hand to grab the elbow then performing lateral flexion (bending side to side). Back extensions can also be performed during this exercise. Perform 3 sets of squats for 10–12 reps then switch.

COMBONATION #3
PULL AND STRETCH

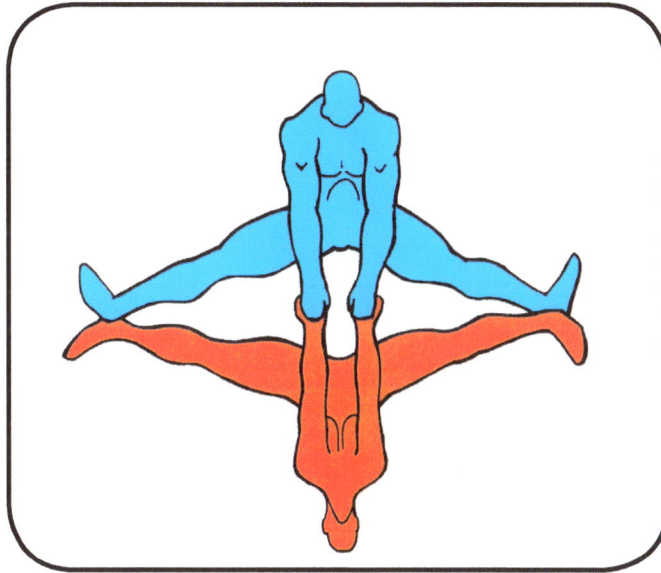

Figure 3-2

Muscles worked:

Legs: Adductor magnus, gracilis, adductor longus, adductor brevis, and pectineus

Back: Latissimus dorsi

The man and woman sit opposite one another, with their legs spread apart and their feet touching. Depending on leg length, the woman's feet may rest on the man's calves or vice versa. Lean forward and clasp hands. Begin by one leaning back and pulling the other forward.

By pulling the upper body forward, the centers come closer together; pushing the legs outward, causing the adductor muscles to stretch, as well as the latissimus dorsi and triceps brachii. Hold each stretch for 5–10 sec. Alternate back and forth for 10–12 reps for 3 sets.

COMBONATION #4
ASSISTED HAMSTRING AND
CALF STRETCH AND MASSAGE

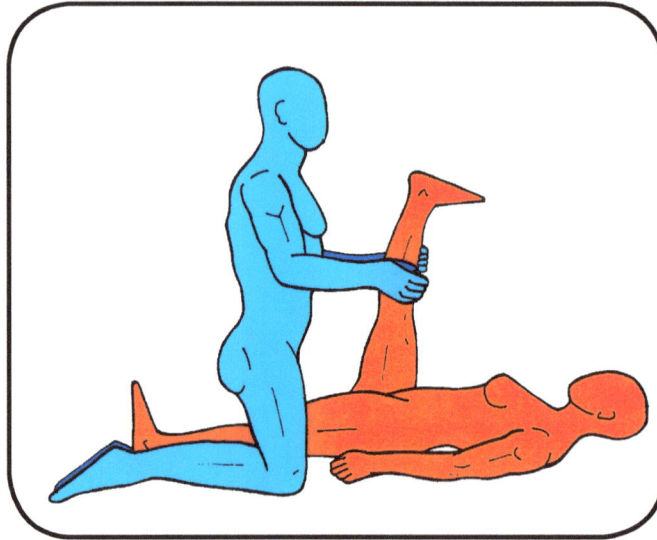

Figure 3-3

Muscles Worked:

Hamstrings: Biceps femoris, semitendinosus, semimembranosus

Calf: Gastrocnemius, soleus

The woman lies in a supine position, with her legs straight, shoulder-width apart, and her arms to her side. The man straddles one of the woman's legs resting on his knees. The woman elevates the free leg until it is perpendicular (90-degrees) to the other, placing it in front of the man.

The man places one hand on the knee and the other on the heel of the foot, slowly and gently assisting in stretching the hamstring. Hold the stretch for 10 seconds then release. Then the man removes his hand from the heel, placing it on the ball of the foot. Then he pulls the foot down, assisting in the dorsiflexion of the woman's foot. Again hold the stretch for 10 seconds and release.

In this position, the man can also perform some massage on the woman's calf and hamstring to further loosen the muscle. When finished, repeat the action on the opposite leg, then switch positions with your partner.

COMBONATION #5
ADDUCTOR STRETCH/BENT LEG
RAISES/DONKEY KICKS

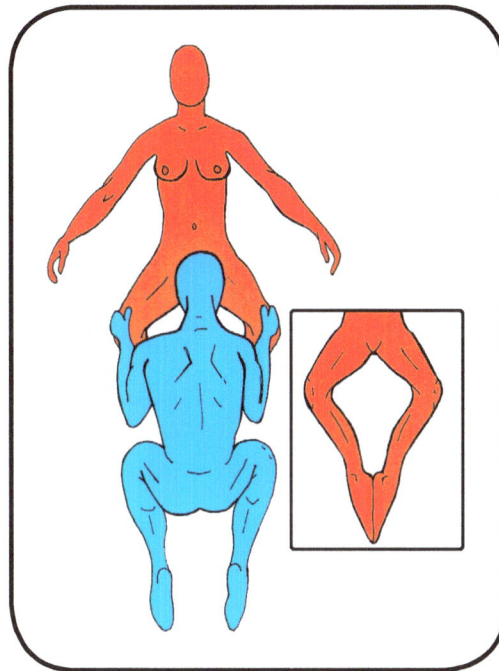

Figure 3-4

Muscles Worked:

Woman: Adductor magnus, gracilis, adductor longus,
adductor brevis, and pectineus

Man: Biceps femoris, semitendinosus, and semimembranosus

The woman lies in the supine position, with the soles of her feet touching, her legs apart, and lowered toward the floor. The man positions himself in front of the woman on his knees, leaning forward, placing his hands or forearms on the woman's knees.

The man applies a small amount of his body weight upon the woman's knees, stretching the adductors. The woman then responds by bringing her legs up or together, by contracting the leg adductors. He can also perform lateral leg raises or bent leg raises. From this position, the woman may also do reps of roll ups, working the middle abdominal muscles. Do any combination of these exercises for 10–15 reps for 3 sets.

CHAPTER FOUR
EXERCISE AND SEX

In chapter 1, we defined what exercise is. In this chapter, we will look at the act of sex and its relationship to exercise. The act of sex is defined as anything connected with sexual gratification or reproduction or the urge for these, especially the attraction of those of one sex for those of the other.

In recent years, there have been more and more studies on the relationship of exercise and sex and how exercise may improve potency. In the Jan/Feb. 2001 issue of *Fitness Matters*, a publication put out by ACE, the American Council on Exercise, an article was written entitled, "Can Exercise Improve Your Sex Life?" Several studies done by leading universities suggest that the answer is yes.

Early in 2001, results from a ten-year Massachusetts Male Aging Study, the largest random sample investigation done to date of Erectile Dysfunction (ED), found a direct correlation between physical inactivity and the lack of sexual potency. Sedentary men had the highest risk for impotence while men who worked out had the lowest.

John McKinlay, an epidemiologist at the New England Research Institute in Watertown, Massachusetts, emphasized that "Of all the lifestyle factors that were considered including quitting cigarettes and alcohol," he says, "the only thing that helped reverse E.D. was taking a brisk walk or the equivalent everyday." Another study, conducted by the Harvard School of Public Health, revealed that men who exercised vigorously for twenty to thirty minutes a day were about half as likely to have erection problems as those who did not. The study also discovered that as a man's waist size increased, so did his chances of becoming an ED candidate.

The University of San Diego did a study of seveny-eight sedentary middle-aged but healthy men proving that those who started working out vigorously (three to four times a week, for sixty minutes per session) reported more frequent sexual activity and orgasms, more reliable function during sex, and a higher percentage of satisfying orgasms.

Exercise isn't a gender-biased sex aid, either; it can help women jump-start their libido, too, says Dr. Cindy Meston, assistant professor of clinical psychology at the University of Texas in Austin. Meston researched thirty-five young women (ages 18–34) who on two separate occasions, watched first a short travel film, then an X-rated film (edited to five minutes in Meston's lab, she says).

The first time, her subjects cycled vigorously for twenty minutes, the second time they didn't. Meston measured their sexual response, using a device that measures blood flow in the genital tissue, and found that after exercising, the women's vaginal responses were 169 percent greater. While they did not compare the differences in fitness levels, Meston says, "it showed that when you do cardio exercise, it not only elevates your blood pressure and heart rate and increases vascularity all over the body, but also seems to facilitate sexual performance." The article goes on and on, quoting numerous doctors and specialist from various fields reporting their findings on the correlation of exercise and sex. This article was a virtual plethora of knowledge, yet with all these findings, we still have tens of millions in this country who are sexually unsatisfied. Therefore exercise alone is not going to improve your sex life.

This brings us back full circle to the definition of sex, which is anything connected with sexual gratification or reproduction or the urge for these, especially the attraction of those of one sex for those of the other.

Sex was meant for the purpose procreation and procreation alone. This is never more evident than in the animal kingdom, where animals mate (have sex) and give birth according to their natural cycle, year in and year out. People, on the other hand, have sex outside of the normal mating cycle for recreational purposes because we are urged by the temptations (appearances) of the opposite sex and are addicted to the sexual gratification (feeling or satisfaction) it has for us. If we are to continue practicing our sexual habits, let us at least use them in a way that might improve our quality of life instead of our social status.

I would like to address the issue of sexual gratification as it relates to our indoctrination of the same as boys and girls. With any issue, I feel it is important to study the historical framework as well as the modern-day perceptions in order to gain a better understanding of the dynamics involved. Sex has always been taboo in our society. As a matter of fact, it is only in recent years that we have openly discussed such issues as sexually transmitted diseases, orgasms, and sexual dysfunction. Because of this yoke and our parents' inability (men in particular) to discuss the duties and responsibilities of the act, most of us were left to be educated by the streets.

As a young man growing up (especially those in the inner city), your manhood is equated to the number of young ladies that you sleep with. Conversely, the length of her virginity and the number of young men she doesn't sleep with determine a young woman's virtue and purity. Allow me to paint a picture for you.

Most often the scenario goes like this: An older sibling or friend instructs you that you must beguile the girls by telling them the things they want and need to hear. This will allow you to fondle their breasts and get into their panties. When you have their clothes off, use such and such positions, twisting the girl's body and legs this way and that way as you thrust as hard as you can.

He further instructs you that satisfaction is not complete until you hear her screaming and moaning and her head is repeatedly hitting the headboard as you're climaxing. This, back then, was affectionately referred to as fucking (Fornication Under the Crown King).

The young ladies, on the other hand, are usually told by their mothers to save themselves for marriage and that special person (in many cases, however, the latter comes before the former) someone who they can give their all to and share everything with—their hopes and dreams and their emotional highs and lows. They are taught some of the virtues of love, so when they do engage in an intimate act, they immediately form an emotional bond.

As you can see, we have two different educational experiences on opposite ends of the continuum. Therein lies the problem of millions that have had or are having bad sexual experiences.

Most men who have not yet honed the ability to control ejaculation or to please a woman do not see their immediate gratification as an issue. But for the women, who require additional attention in order to reach orgasm, this is an issue of great concern.

In order to undo years of miseducation, we must first learn to understand our partner's mind-set by openly communicating and appreciating the others needs and desires.

Some wise man once said that you must first learn the past in order to understand the present to know where you're going in the future. Now that we have a better idea of where we came from and where we are at present, the future should be much more fulfilling. I believe we are now ready to get into the meat of the exercise program itself.

The following are a series of exercises designed to target the major muscle groups. Some combonations are best performed during foreplay and others during the act of intimacy. There are many methods of training; some are better than others. It just depends on the fitness professional or fitness magazine you choose to follow. Some say superslow sets are the best method, others prefer active recovery, and still others recommend super sets. Though their methods may vary, most fitness professionals will agree that the major (larger) muscle groups (chest, back, and legs) should be targeted first to prevent expending unnecessary energy on the secondary muscle groups (arms, shoulders, abs).

First we will begin with the *Chest*. Figures 4-1 and 4-2 combonations on pages 32 and 33 respectively demonstrate two variations of female push-ups and the man working the middle and side abdominal muscles. Figures 4-3 through 4-5 on pages 34 through 36 demonstrate the man doing push-ups as the woman performs the pelvic thrust, crunches, and roll ups respectively. Figures 4-6 through 4-9 on pages 37 through 40 are for the more advanced fitness person. These exercises require higher degrees of strength and coordination. *Do not* attempt to perform these exercises if you are at the novice or intermediate levels. Failure to follow these instructions may result in serious injuries.

COMBONATION #6
TORSO TWIST AND PUSH-UPS

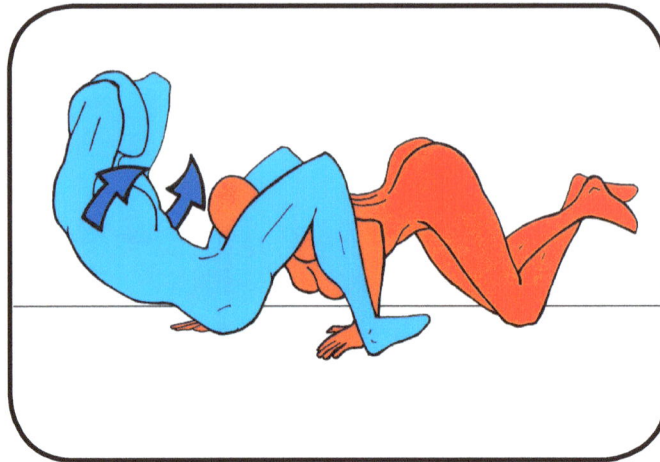

Figure 4-1

Muscles Worked:
Man: Internal and external obliques
Woman: Pectoralis major and triceps brachii

The man lies in a supine position, with his legs apart, bent at a 45-degree angle, placing his hands to the side of his head. The woman positions herself on her knees between his legs.

Using a twisting action, the man rises up, bringing his elbow to the knee of the opposite side, first working the internal obliques. He then rotates, bringing the other elbow to the opposite knee, working the external obliques, contracting for 2–3 seconds. He then lowers himself back to the mat.

The woman performs push-ups in one of three ways: 1) female style as depicted in the illustration. 2) modified, placing the feet approximately shoulder-width apart, which increases stability. 3) advanced, placing one leg over top of the other, causing you to use more upper body to stabilize yourself.

As the man rises to the up position of the sit-up, the woman should lower herself to the concentric or downward position of the push-up, which will allow her to kiss or lick his inner thigh as well as orally massage his penis. Do 10–15 reps for 3 sets.

COMBONATION #7
CRUNCHES AND PUSH-UPS

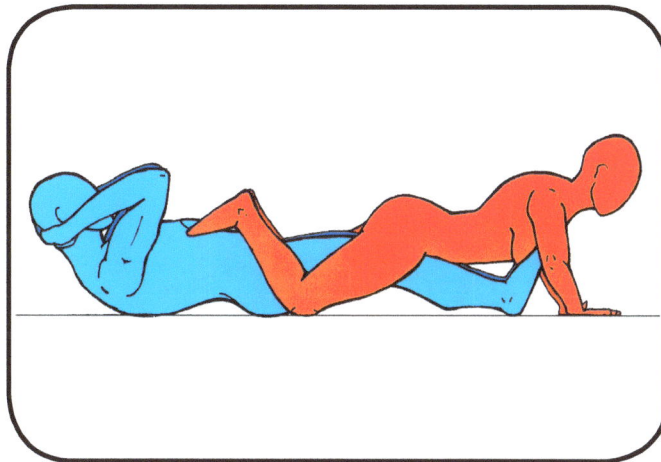

Figure 4-2

Muscles Worked:

Man: Rectus abdominis

Woman: Pectoralis major, triceps brachii

The man lies in a supine position, with his legs slightly bent and apart, placing his hands to the side of his head. The woman straddles the man's lower thighs, positioning herself on her hands and knees.

The man rises up, performing roll ups, contracting the abdominal muscles for 2–3 seconds, then releasing and lowering himself back to the mat.

The woman performs push-ups in one of two ways: 1) female style as depicted in the illustration, or 2) modified, placing the toes on the floor approximately shoulder-width apart, providing greater stability.

As the man rises to the up position of the roll up for 20–30 reps, he will view the posterior anatomy of his partner. The woman on the other hand, performs the push-ups for 10–15 reps, enticing and arousing her intimate onlooker. Do 3 sets.

COMBONATION #8
PUSH-UPS AND TUSH TIGHTENERS

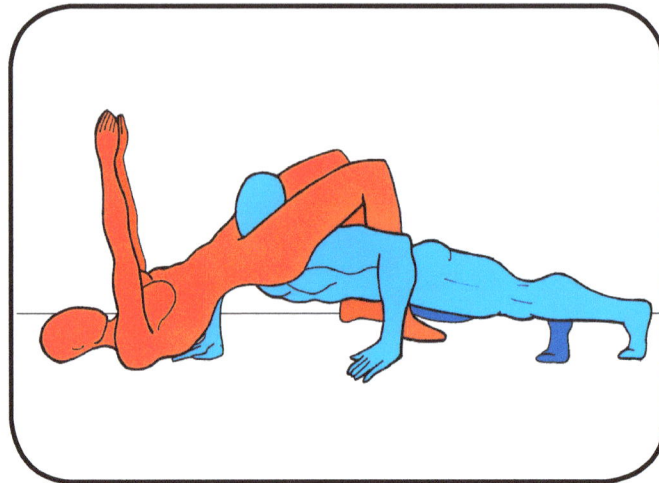

Figure 4-3

Muscles Worked:

Men: Pectoralis major and triceps brachii

Women: Pubococcygeus, gluteus, and hip rotators

The woman lies in a supine position, with her legs shoulder-width apart, bent at a 45-degree angle, and her arms to her side. The man lies down between her legs in a push-up position.

The woman raises her buttocks off the mat, performing the tush tightener, squeezing her buttocks tightly for 1–3 seconds then releasing and lowering herself to the mat. The squeezing action can also indirectly work the pubococcygeus, or PC, muscles. These are the muscles used to prevent urination.

When she raises her buttocks, the man will rise with her at the same rate of speed, bringing him to the up position of the push-up. From the lower position to the up position, the man should suck gently on her clitoris, stopping to breathe on the downward motion. This oral stimulus will enhance the muscle contraction of the tush tightener since a woman often assumes this position during orgasm. Do 10–15 reps for 3 sets.

COMBONATION #9
PUSH-UPS AND CRUNCHES

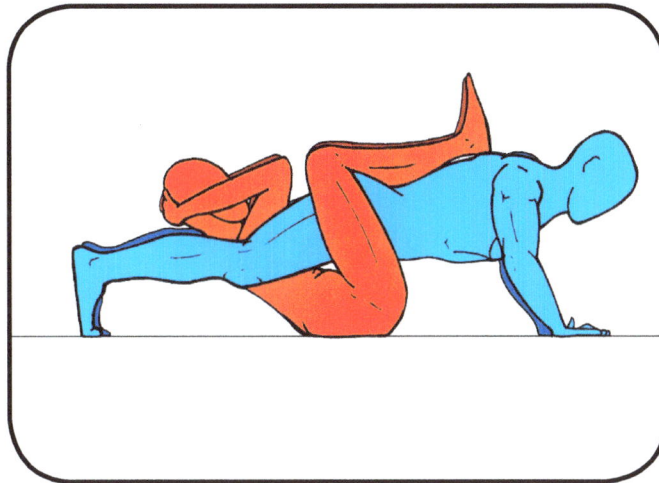

Figure 4-4

Muscles Worked:
Man: Pectoralis major, triceps brachii, and anterior deltoid
Woman: Rectus abdominis

The woman lies in a supine position, with her hands to the sides of her head, legs apart and elevated in the air. The man faces away from the woman, straddles her, and lowers himself down between her legs and onto his knees and forearms.

From this inverted angle, he penetrates the woman then assumes the push-up position. Performing the push-up in this position will greatly change the angle and depth of penetration. While the man performs the push-up exercise, the woman will engage in crunches, working the middle and upper abdominal region. Do 10–15 reps for 3 sets.

COMBONATION #10
CRUNCHES AND PUSH-UP

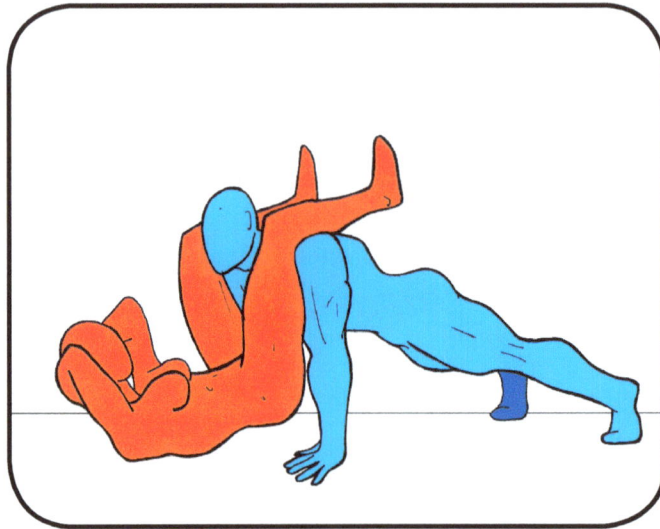

Figure 4-5

Muscles Worked:
Man: Pectoralis major, anterior deltiod, triceps brachii
Woman: Rectus abdominis * internal and external obliques

The woman lies in a supine position, with her hands to the sides of her head, legs apart and elevated in the air, waiting to receive the man. The man situates himself in front of the woman and assumes the push-up position, with his head between her thighs and her calves over his shoulder blades.

This is a more advanced combonation in that the man has increased resistance due to the woman placing her legs over his shoulders. She performs crunches when he is in the upward phase of the push-up.

*Also, she may work the internal and external obliques by pointing her elbows to the opposite knee. Do 10–15 reps for 3 sets.

COMBONATION #11
WALL PUSH-UPS AND MASSAGE

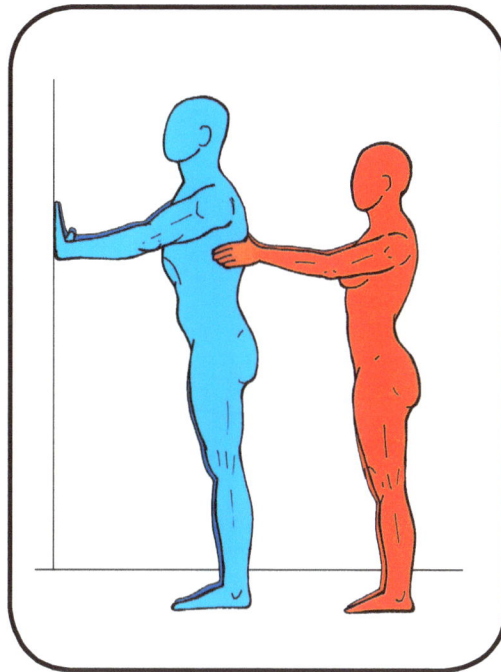

Figure 4-6

Muscles Worked:

Man: Pectoralis major, anterior deltoid, serratus
anterior, and triceps brachii

Muscles Massaged:

Woman: Levator scapulae, trapezius, rhomboids,
erector spinae, and quadratus lumborum

The man stands upright, 3–4 feet away from the wall, then leans forward, placing his hands on the wall. The woman stands behind the man, with her hands placed on his shoulder blades (hand placement may vary), applying force, which will act as the resistance for the man.

The man begins by lowering himself closer to the wall then pushing away, performing the chest press, while the woman applies force on his back and massages the working muscles. Do 10–15 reps for 3 sets.

COMBONATION #12
PUSH-UPS AND CRUNCHES

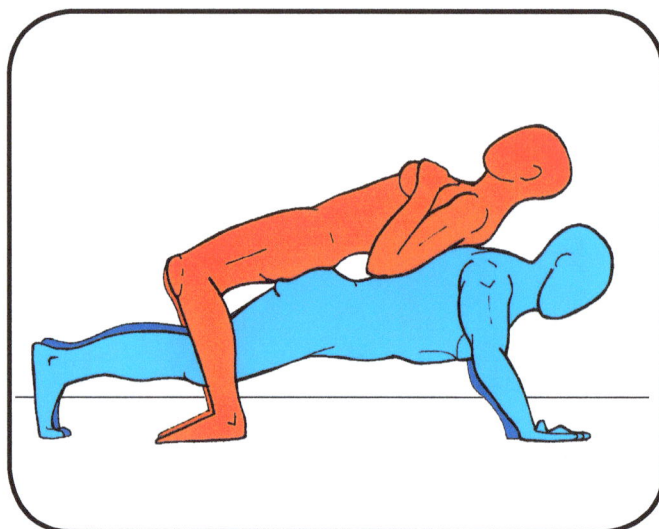

Figure 4-7

Muscles Worked:

Man: Pectoralis major, anterior deltoids, triceps brachii

Woman: Rectus abdominis

The man lowers himself to the mat and assumes the up phase of the push-up. The woman faces away from the man. She straddles him and lies in a supine position on his back. The woman's body weight adds to the resistance of the exercise while the man performs push-ups. When the man is in the down phase, the woman will perform roll ups similar to those performed on a Swiss ball. This is an advanced combonation that has definite strength requirements. Do 5–10 reps. for 2–3 sets.

COMBONATION #13
PUSH-UPS AND CHEST PRESS

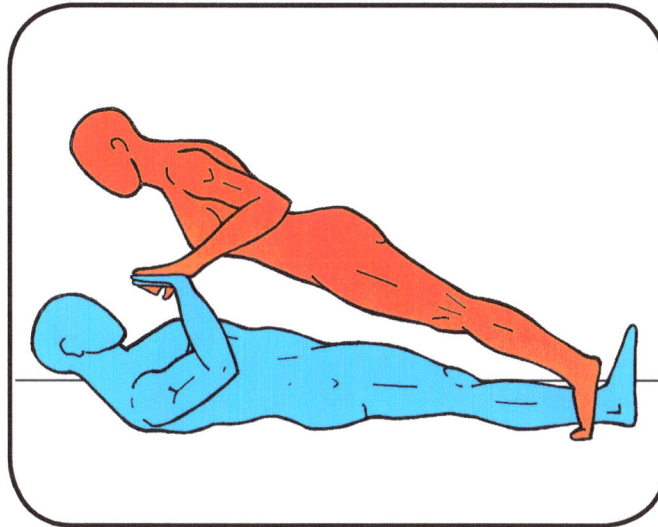

Figure 4-8

Muscles Worked: (Man and Woman)
Pectoralis major and triceps brachii

The man lies in a supine position, with his legs together and his arms stretched upward. The woman stands atop the man with her legs approximately shoulder-width apart for stability. She then leans forward, placing her hands onto the palms of the man, interlacing his fingers.

The man lowers the woman by performing the eccentric (negative) motion of the bench press. The woman lowers herself performing the eccentric motion of the push-up. She then pushes away doing the concentric (positive) motion of the push-up, as does the man with the chest press. This is an advanced combonation that requires strength and coordination. Do 5–10 reps for 2–3 sets.

COMBONATION #14
PUSH-UPS AND PELVIC THRUSTS

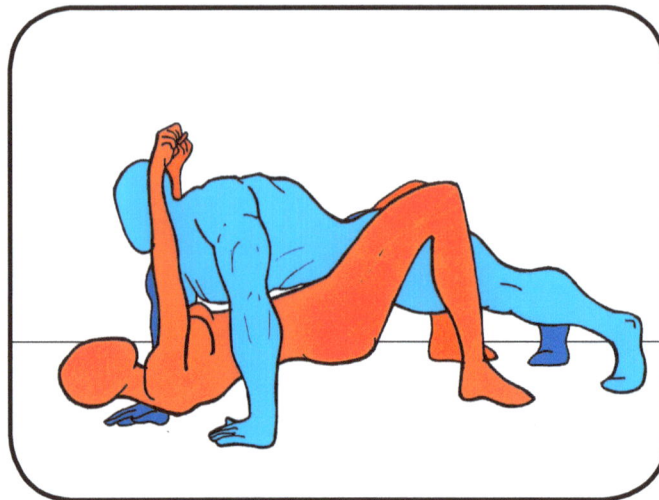

Figure 4-9

Muscles Worked:
Man: Pectoralis major, Anterior deltoid
Woman: Lower rectus abdominis

The woman lies in a supine position, with her legs apart, bent at a 45-degree angle. The man positions himself to penetrate and assumes the down phase of the push-up exercise. The man rises slowly to the up phase, supporting the majority of his body weight with his upper body while placing approximately 20–30 percent of his weight across her pelvic region.

The woman begins to perform the pelvic thrust by lifting her buttocks off the mat, working the lower abdominal muscles, using the man's body weight as the resistance. She holds this position for 2–3 seconds, contracting the abdominal muscles, then lowers her buttocks back to the mat as the man also returns to his starting position. Do 10–12 reps for 3 sets.

The next muscle group is the **Back**. Be aware that all exercises should be done in an opposing nature, meaning that when you work your chest, you should work your back in the next workout session. This is a type of homeostasis, which keeps the muscle groups in proper balance. Figures 4-10 through 4-13 combonations on pages 41 through 44 respectfully demonstrate reciprocating lawnmower pulls, reverse flies, lat pull downs, and sharks

COMBONATION #15
REVERSE FLIES AND CHEST FLIES

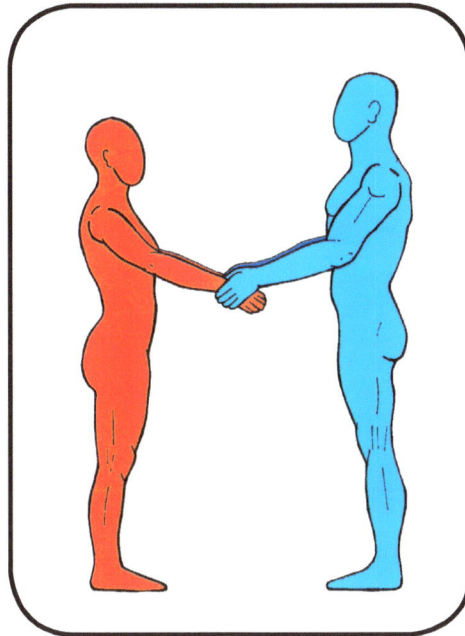

Figure 4-10

Muscles Worked:

Man: Pectoralis major

Woman: Rhomboids, middle trapezius, posterior deltoid

The man and woman stand in an upright posture, facing one another, their feet shoulder-width apart, with a distance of approximately two feet between them. Both the man and woman extend their arms out in front until they are perpendicular to the floor.

The man places his hands on the anterior (top) side of the woman's hands. The woman then attempts to open her arms laterally, performing the concentric (positive) contraction of the reverse fly. The man, on the other hand, offers resistance by performing the eccentric (negative) contraction of the chest fly.

The man will then attempt to close his hands, performing the concentric action of the chest fly, while the woman offers resistance as she performs the eccentric action of the reverse fly. Do 10–15 reps for 3 sets.

COMBONATION #16
RECIPROCATING LAWNMOWER PULLS

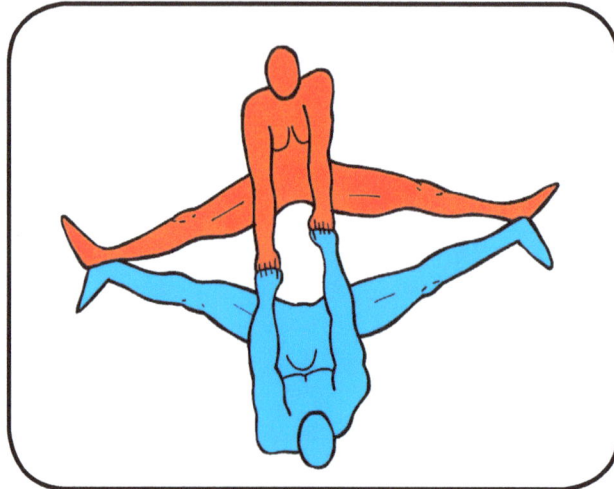

Figure 4-11

Muscles Worked:
Back: Latissimus dorsi
*****Legs**: Adductor magnus, gracilis, adductor longus,
adductor brevis, pectineus

The man and woman sit opposite one another, holding hands, with their legs spread apart and their feet touching. Depending on the length of the woman's legs, her feet may rest on the man's calves. The man begins the exercise by bringing one arm close to his body, performing the concentric action of the lawnmower pull.

The woman, on the other hand, offers resistance by performing the eccentric action of the lawnmower pull. Then, using the opposite hand, the woman draws her hand close to her body, performing the concentric action as the man now offers resistance by performing the eccentric action.

*This combonation will also allow you to stretch the leg muscles as it is similar to the exercise in figure 3-2. By one of you leaning back and pulling the other forward, your centers will naturally come closer together, pushing the legs outward, causing the adductor muscles to stretch. Alternate back and forth for 10–12 reps and for 3 sets.

COMBONATION #17
BUTTERFLIES

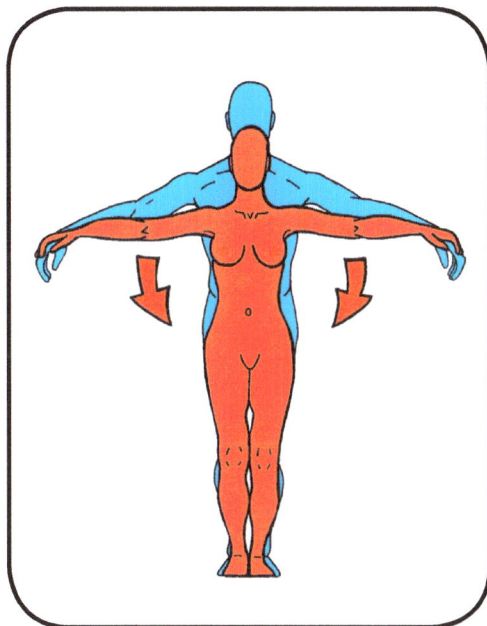

Figure 4-12

Muscles Worked:
Man: Lateral deltoids
Woman: Latissimus dorsi and teres major

The man and woman stand in an upright posture, with the woman pressing her posterior (backside) against the man's anterior (front). With their hands to their sides, the woman places her hand on the anterior side of the man's hands.

The man then attempts to raise his arms up to the perpendicular position, performing the concentric action of the lateral dumbbell raise. The woman then offers resistance by opposing his action while performing the eccentric action of the iron cross.

After your arms are parallel to the floor, the woman then attempts to lower her arms, performing the concentric action of the iron cross while the man offers resistance by performing the eccentric action of the lateral dumbbell raise. Do 10–15 reps for 3 sets.

COMBONATION #18
SHARKS

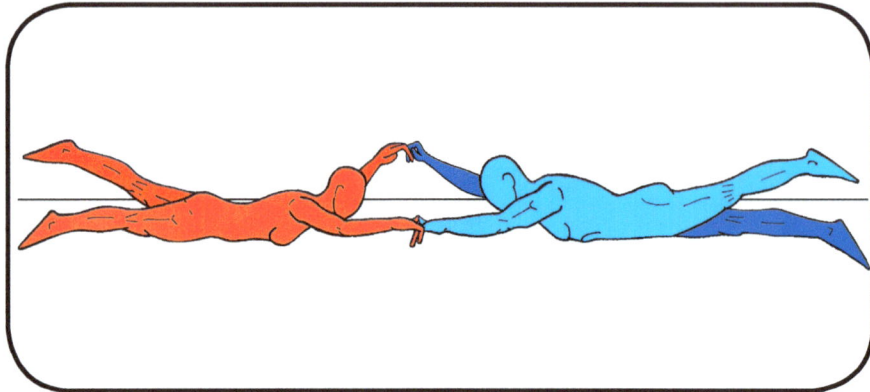

Figure 4-13

Muscles Worked: (Man and Woman) Biceps femoris,
semitendinosus, semimembranosus, gluteus maximus,
erector spinae group, and transversospinalis group

Both the man and woman lie facing one another in a prone (on belly) position, with their arms extended, fingers interlaced, and their toes pointed. Pretending to be in shark-infested waters and having to swim to shore, the man raises his right arm and left leg. The woman raises her left arm and right leg simultaneously. They lower their respective extremities simultaneously and raise the others in the same manner repetitiously, causing a swimming effect. Perform this exercise for 15–30 seconds, rest, and then repeat the action 3–5 times.

By now it should be obvious that most of these exercises can be performed individually, but they become much more interesting with a partner who you have a deep appreciation for. Working as a team helps to build unity through trust and communication. It also gives you a support unit to pull you through those tough times and to spur you on on those days you just don't feel like doing anything. Through thick and thin—does that sound familiar? Let us continue.

The next muscle group is the **Arms** (biceps and triceps). Figures 4-14 through 4-17 on pages 45 through 48 demonstrate biceps curls and triceps extensions.

COMBONATION #19
BICEPS CURL AND TRICEPS EXTENSIONS

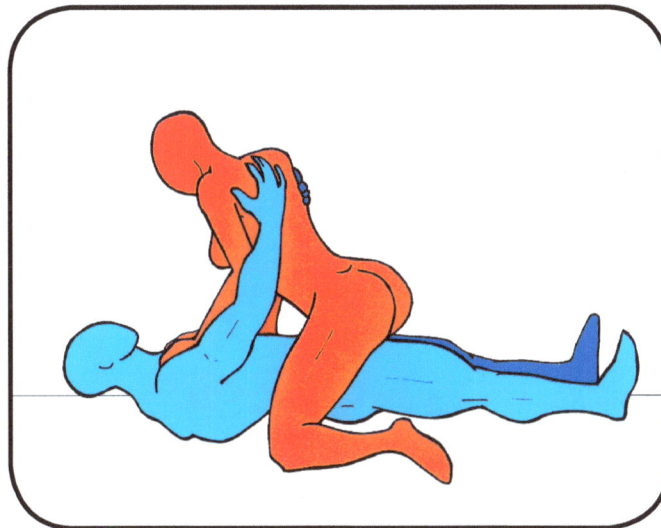

Figure 4-14

Muscles Worked:

Man: Biceps brachii, brachialis, brachioradialis

Woman: Triceps brachii

The man lies in a supine position. The woman straddles the man and lowers herself to a kneeling position, inserting his penis into her vagina. He then puts his arms under her axillary (armpit) area, placing his hands onto her scapula area (shoulder blades). She places her hands onto his chest. During intercourse, tell her to offer some resistance, but do not lock elbows. When she does this, pull her toward you until you are face to face.

This action simulates the concentric (positive) contraction of the biceps curl. For the woman, the action will simulate the eccentric (negative) contraction of the triceps extension. Reward each other with a kiss, then have her push away as you offer resistance by holding her close, but not too tight. This action will provide the negative contraction of the biceps curl while providing the positive contraction of the triceps extension. Do 10–15 reps for 3 sets.

COMBONATION #20
TRICEPS EXTENSION AND BICEPS CURL

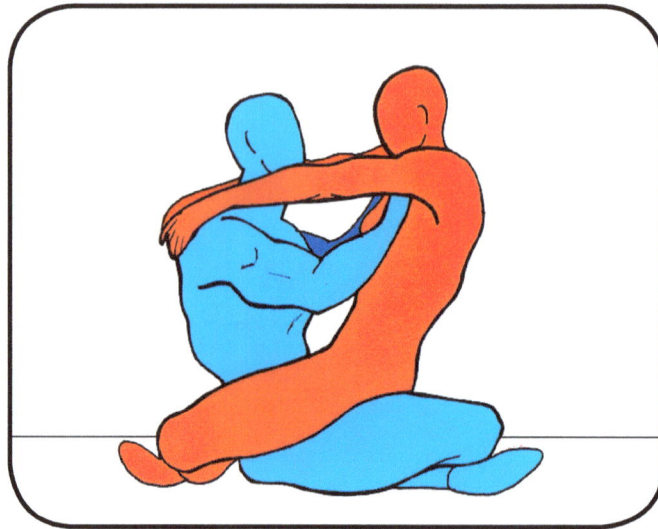

Figure 4-15

Muscles Worked:
Man: Triceps brachii
Woman: Biceps brachii, brachialis, and brachioradialis

The man sits down in an Indian-style position or modified position, depending on your comfort level. The woman then straddles the man, lowering herself onto the penis, inserting it into the vagina. In this position, the man will work his triceps by placing his hands on the upper portion of the woman's chest, pushing her away as she offers resistance, simulating the concentric (positive) action of the triceps extension.

With her hands placed on either the lateral portion of the deltoids (shoulders) or under the axillary (armpit) area and onto the scapulas (shoulder blades), the woman will simulate the eccentric (negative) action of the biceps curl. When the woman attempts to pull him close, she is performing the concentric (positive) action of the curl. He on the other hand would be performing the eccentric (negative) action of the tricep extension. When face to face, kiss for a few seconds, then repeat the action. Do this 10–15 reps for 3 sets.

COMBONATION #21
TORSO TWIST AND TRICEPS

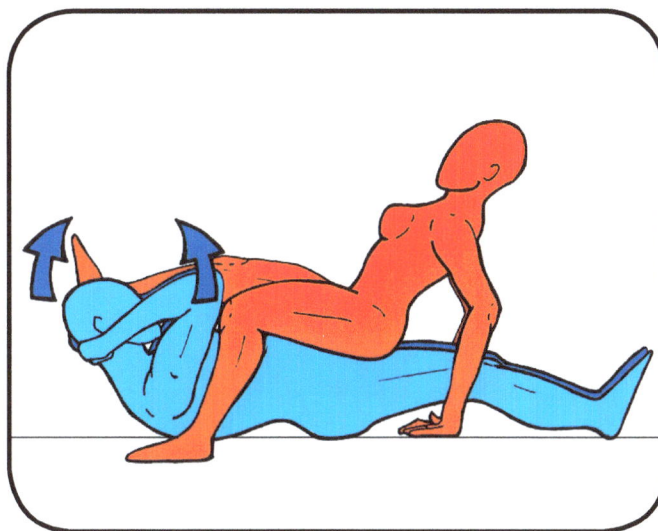

Figure 4-16

Muscles Worked:
Man: Internal obliques
Woman: Biceps brachii

The man lies in a supine position, with his legs together, slightly bent, and his hands to the sides of his head. The woman faces the man, straddles him, and lowers herself, inserting his penis into her vagina. Placing her hands on the mat, the woman leans back and bends at the elbow, lowering herself, then pushes up, working the tricep muscles. Depending on strength and comfort level, the woman can elevate her legs in the air, increasing depth of penetration and exercise difficulty.

The man rolls up, working the rectus abdominis muscles. He pauses, then points one elbow to the opposite knee, contracting the internal obliques. Maintaining this position for 1 second, he then returns to the up position and lowers himself back to the mat. Holding this position will help to build muscle endurance as well as muscle tone. Do this for 10–12 reps for 3 sets.

COMBONATION #22
DIP AND SQUATS

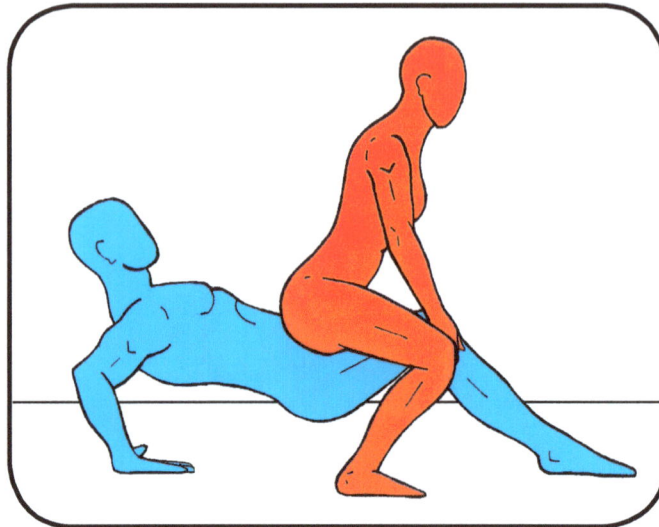

Figure 4-17

Muscles Worked:

Man: Triceps brachii

Woman: Quadriceps femoris and gluteus maximus

The man sits on his buttocks, with his knees bent slightly less than 45-degrees. Leaning back, he places his hands on the mat, shoulder-width apart. The woman faces away from the man and straddles him, lowering herself onto his penis and inserting it into the vagina. The woman rises a few inches, allowing the man to come up to the starting position. Keeping his buttocks off the mat, the man begins to bend at the elbows, dipping down, causing the eccentric (negative) contraction. He then pushes upward, which is the concentric (positive) contraction of the dip. The woman, meanwhile, rides the wave using her legs to rise up and down, doing hack squats and stabilizing her posture. Do 10–15 reps for 3 sets.

Moving on to the *Shoulders* brings us to several combonations that offer couples an intimate embrace. Touch is a very important part of our existence as creatures of nature. To fully understand this concept, observe an owner of an animal as he or she pets the animal. Notice how calm and secure that animal appears in the embrace of his owner. The same can be said for a person who needs to be touched.

In the book *The Five Love Languages: How to Express Heartfelt Commitment to Your Mate*, by Gary Chapman, Ph.D., the author states that physical touch can make or break a relationship. It can communicate hate or love. I agree with him 100% on this point and recommend this book to all couples.

As a massage therapist, I have an appreciation for the sense of touch for both its psychological and therapeutic benefits. Figures 4-18 and 4-19 on pages 50 and 51 demonstrate exercises for the anterior and lateral deltoid muscles that bring couples close together, allowing them to embrace at the end of the set. Figure 4-12 on page 43 can also be included in the shoulder routine.

COMBONATION #23
FRONTAL SHOULDER RAISES AND
LATISSIMUS DORSI PULL DOWN

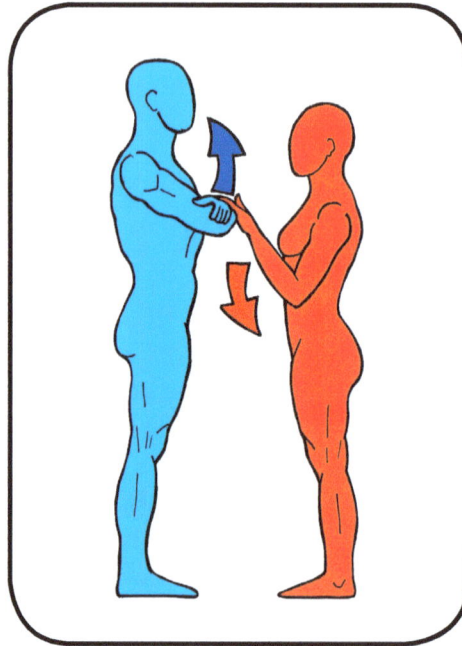

Figure 4-18

Muscles Worked:

Man: Anterior deltoid and biceps brachii

Woman: Latissimus dorsi, teres major, and biceps brachii (small head)

The man and woman stand in an upright posture, facing one another with their feet shoulder-width apart, with a distance of approximately two feet between them. The man folds his arms while the woman places her hands on the inside of his elbows. The man elevates his arms to a perpendicular position, performing the concentric (positive) action of the frontal dumbbell raise.

The woman offers resistance by performing the eccentric (negative) action of the latissimus pull down. She then attempts to lower her arms, performing the concentric action of the latissimus pull down while the man then offers resistance by performing the eccentric action of the frontal dumbbell raise. Do 10–15 reps for 3 sets.

COMBONATION #24
LATERAL SHRUGS AND LATISSIMUS FLIES

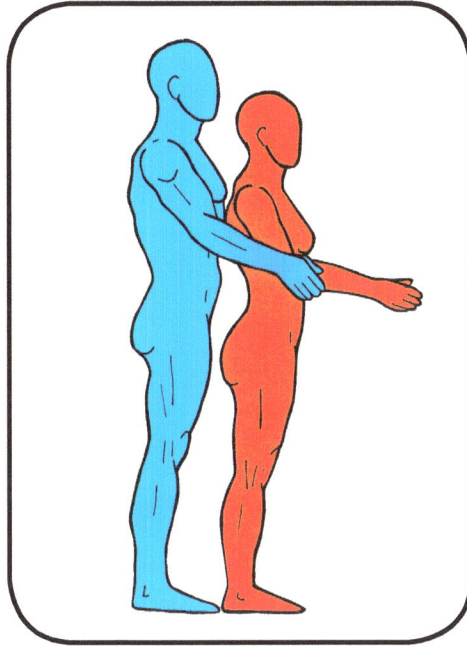

Figure 4-19

Muscles Worked:
Man: Latissimus dorsi and teres major
Woman: Middle deltoid, supraspinatus, and upper trapezius

The man stands in an upright posture, with his arms to his side while the woman positions herself in front of him, pressing her posterior (buttocks) against his penis. The woman bends her arms to a 90-degree angle at the elbow, with the man placing his hands on top of her arms at the elbow.

While embraced, the woman attempts to raise her arms laterally, performing the concentric (positive) action of the lateral shoulder shrug. The man, meanwhile, offers resistance by performing the eccentric (negative) action of the latissimus fly. During the concentric phase of the latissimus fly, the man attempts to lower his arms while the woman offers resistance by performing the eccentric phase of the lateral shoulder shrug. Do 10–15 reps for 3 sets.

Note: Changing the placement of the hands will vary the degree of resistance. Now let's move to the lower extremities, the **Legs**, which make up our foundation and base of support. Most of the exercises illustrated can be performed during the act of intimacy. It is important to have strong legs since they do the brunt of the work during the day while transporting you from place to place. Research shows that more testosterone is released while working the leg group than any other muscle group. Testosterone is the male sex hormone, so it would stand to reason that if more testosterone were released, the libido would be more active. This would be very beneficial to the man.

Though the woman possesses lower levels of testosterone and I have not heard of any such increase of the same, I have observed that women with firm butts and shapely legs feel much sexier and more confident about their appearance.

Figures 4-20 through 4-26 on pages 53 through 59 demonstrate several exercises targeting the problem areas for women and some strengthening exercises for men.

COMBONATION #25
CALF RAISES

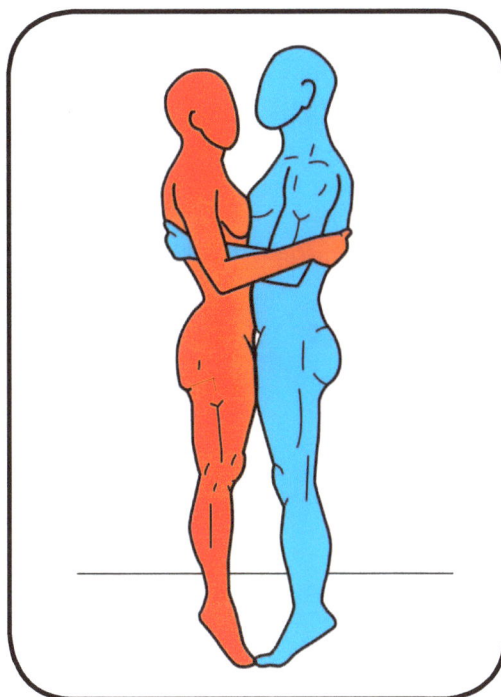

Figure 4-20

Muscles Worked:

Man and Woman Gastrocnemius, soleus,
peroneus brevis, and peroneus longus

Both the man and the woman stand facing one another, embraced in a hug or placing their hands on each another's midriff sections in an intimate fashion to stabilize one another. In unison, both the man and woman rise up on their toes, contracting the calf muscles. Hold for 1–2 seconds then release. This is a great opportunity to look into each other's eyes, kiss, hug, and touch one another. Do these 10–15 reps for 3 sets.

COMBONATION #26
DONKEY KICK AND TORSO TWIST

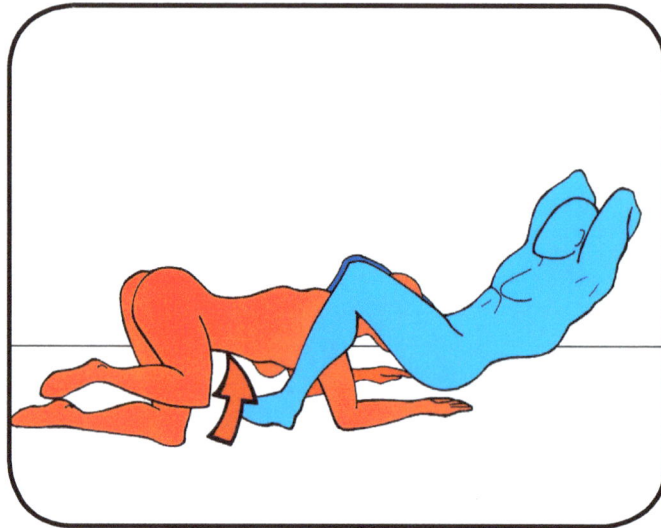

Figure 4-21

Muscles Worked:
Man: External and internal oblique
Woman: Gluteus medius and minimus

The man lies on his back in a supine position, with his legs apart and bent at a 45-degree angle. He then places his hands to the sides of his head, with his elbows pointed outward. The woman positions herself, on her forearms and knees, between his legs. The man will rise up, bringing the left elbow toward the right knee, and return to the mat. He rises again, this time bringing the right elbow toward the left knee, then returns to the mat. This will work the internal and external obliques.

As the man performs the torso twist, the woman performs donkey kicks, raising her leg laterally (outward), keeping it bent at a 45-degree angle, working one side at a time. As she works the hip abductors she can kiss and lick his inner thigh, making her way to his penis, creating an incredible oral stimulus. The man can perform between 10–30 reps and the woman, 10–15 reps for 3 sets.

COMBONATION #27
PONY RIDE AND ROLL UPS

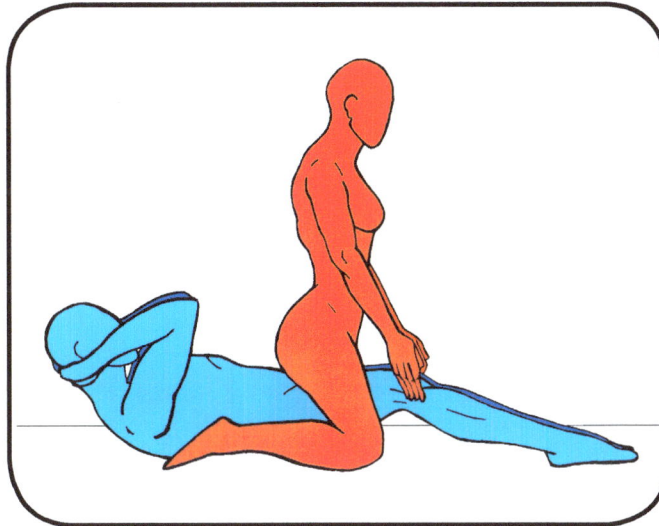

Figure 4-22

Muscles Worked:

Man: Internal and external obliques

Woman: Adductor magnus, adductor longus, adductor brevis, and pectineus

The man lies in a supine position, with his hands to the sides of his head and his legs together, bent at a slight angle. The woman faces away from the man, straddles him, and lowers herself to her knees, allowing the penis to penetrate the vagina. The man rises up, pointing the left elbow to the right knee, lowers himself, and repeats the action to the opposite side. The woman slides her legs apart, then uses the adductor muscles to bring them back. This allows the woman to control the depth and rate of penetration. Do 10–15 reps for 3 sets.

COMBONATION #28
ROLL UPS AND ADDUCTORS SQUATS/STRETCHES

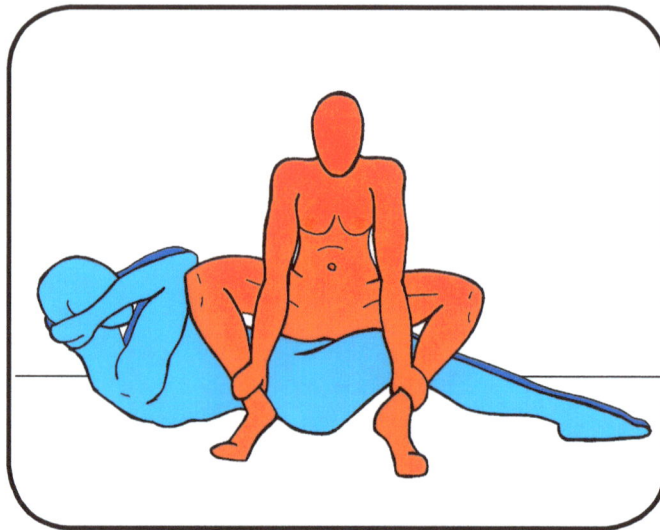

Figure 4-23

Muscles Worked:

Man: Rectus abdominis

Woman: Quadriceps femoris group and gluteus maximus

The man lies in a supine position, with his hands to the sides of his head, legs together, and bent at a slight angle. The woman straddles the man (this can be done from multiple angles) and lowers herself, allowing the penis to penetrate the vagina. The woman performs squats from this position, controlling the depth of penetration.

Between sets of squats the woman leans forward, placing her hands around her ankles and her elbows against her knees, and begins to push outward, stretching the groin or adductor muscles. The man will perform roll ups, rising up, contracting the abdominal muscles for 1–2 seconds, targeting the middle and upper rectus abdominis, then returning back to the mat. Do 10–15 reps for 3 sets.

COMBONATION #29
PARTIAL SIT-UPS AND BENT KNEE EXTENSIONS

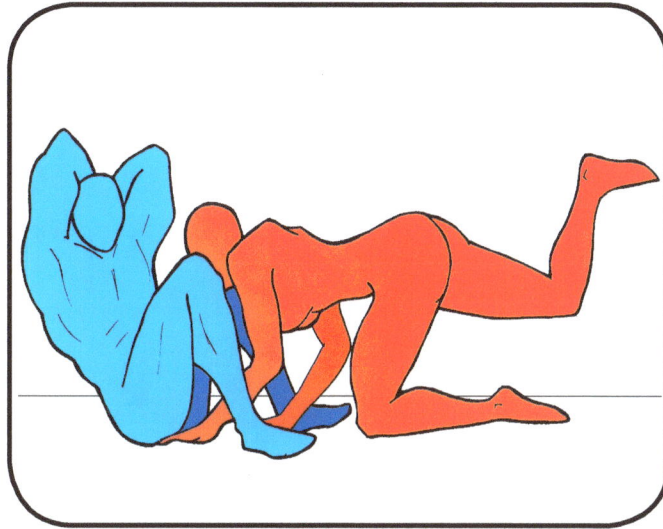

Figure 4-24

Muscles Worked:

Man: Rectus abdominis and transverse abdominis

Woman: Biceps femoris, semitendinosus,

semimembranosus and gluteus maximus

The man lies in a supine position, with his legs apart, bent at a 45-degree angle, and his arms to his side. The woman positions herself on her hands and knees between his legs. From this position, the man will rise up, doing a partial sit-up, working on the middle section of the abdominal region, holding for 1–2 seconds, releasing, and lower himself to the mat.

The woman will perform bent-knee extensions, raising her leg up, keeping it to a 90-degree angle, holding for 1–2 seconds, then releasing. While doing the bent knee extension, she can and should kiss, lick, or blow on his inner thigh, working her way down to the penis, providing an oral stimulus which will divert some of the focus from the working muscle group. The man should do between 10–20 sit-ups, and the woman should do between 10–15 reps per leg for 3 sets.

COMBONATION #30
HACK SQUATS AND MASSAGE

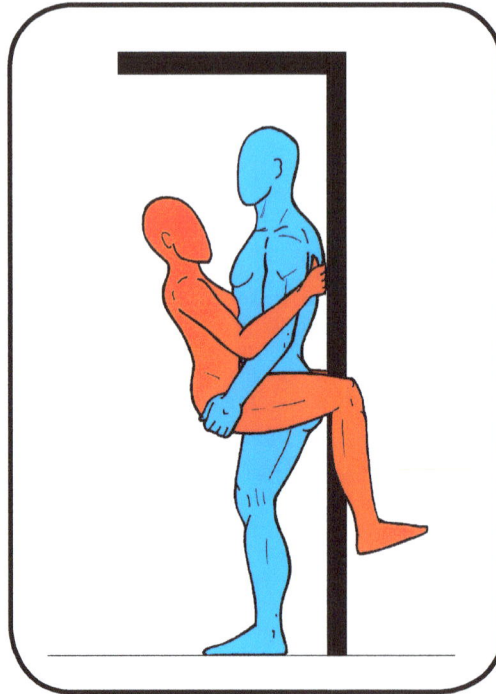

Figure 4-25

Muscles Worked:

Man: Quadriceps femoris group and gluteus maximus

Woman's Massage: Upper trapezius, anterior, lateral, and posterior deltoids, and pectoralis major

The man stands in a doorway, with his feet shoulder-width apart, leaning back against the doorjamb for support and stability. The woman stands directly in front of the man, with her legs apart and her hands on his shoulder. The man then bends at the knees, placing his hand under the woman's thighs, lifting her up to the ready position. The woman takes her hand, places it on the penis, and inserts it into the vagina, then places the hand back on the shoulder area.

The man begins to perform the hack squat by bending at the knees, and lowering himself to a half-squat position, then pushing up, returning to the start position. This also changes the angle and depth of penetration. The woman, meanwhile, massages the shoulders, arms, and chest areas of the man. Do 5–10 reps for 2-3 sets.

COMBONATION #31
HACK SQUATS AND MASSAGE (VARIATION)

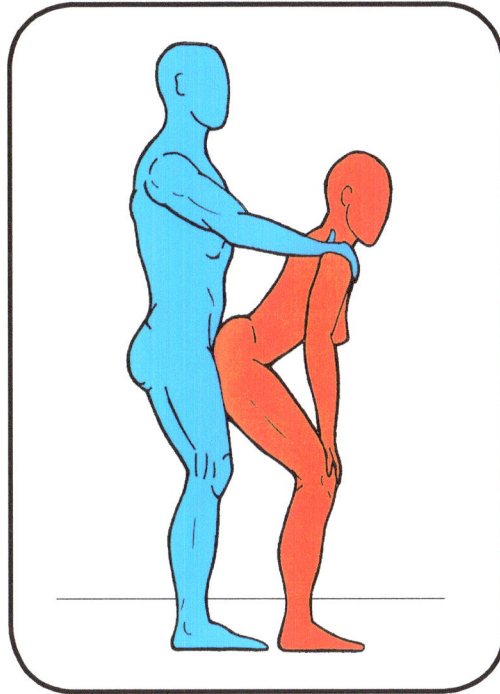

Figure 4-26

Muscles Worked:

Man and Woman: Quadriceps femoris and Gluteus maximus

Massage: Anterior, lateral, and posterior deltoids,
trapezius, and rhomboids

The man stands upright, with his feet shoulder-width apart, placing his hands on the woman's shoulders. She is positioned in front of him with her knees bent, hands on thighs, and her buttocks pressed against his penis. Depending on the height difference, the man may penetrate the woman from behind.

The woman gyrates back and forth, up and down, against the man's penis, working on the quadriceps femoris muscles. The man may also mirror the woman's movements, changing the angle and depth of penetration while massaging the woman's shoulders, trapezius, and rhomboid areas. Do 10–15 reps for 2–3 sets.

We have now reached the most targeted and the most difficult muscle group to work on: the **Abdomen**. The abdomen actually consists of four individual muscle groups: rectus abdominis, external oblique, internal oblique, and the transverse abdominis. The muscle fibers in each group go in different directions to help stabilize the torso.

Strong abdominal muscles must be accompanied by strong back muscles and vice versa because if these groups are unbalanced, it will have an effect on your posture. Understand that when you contract the stomach muscles, you are also stretching the back muscles, and if this were to persist without strengthening the back muscles, it would appear as if you had a bulge when in fact you have strong abdomen muscles. This is the importance of opposing exercises. So remember that when you work your triceps, you must work your biceps, and if you work your quadriceps, then you must work your hamstrings, etc.

Many of the combonations presented thus far incorporated some form of abdominal exercise. The following illustrations, figures 4-27 through 4-29 on pages 61 through 63, are exercises geared specifically for abdominal muscles that couples can do in unison.

COMBONATION #32
FOUR-COUNT LEG LIFTS

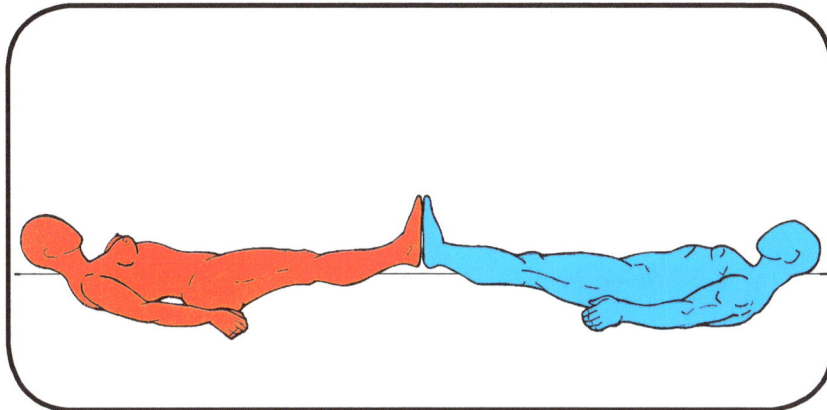

Figure 4-27

Muscles Worked:

Man and Woman: Rectus abdominus, iliopsoas, and rectus femoris

Both the man and woman lie down in a supine position opposite one another, with the soles of their feet touching and their hands under their buttocks. Working together as a team, they should maintain a six-inch distance between the floor and their heels. They begin by: (1) raising their legs off the ground, (2) spreading their legs apart, (3) bringing their legs back together, and (4) lowering their legs back to the starting or resting position.

To increase the level of difficulty, you may pause and maintain each step for a few additional seconds before moving on to the next. Be sure to count aloud in unison. Repeat steps 1 through 4 for 10–15 reps for 3 sets.

COMBONATION #33
BICYCLING

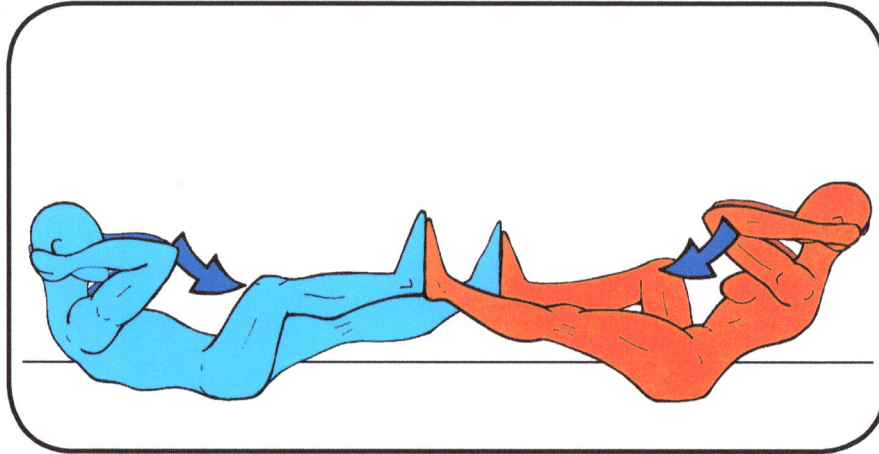

Figure 4-28

Muscles Worked:

Man and Woman: Internal and external obliques

Both the man and woman lie in a supine position opposite one another, with the soles of their feet touching. Coming close enough together, their legs should be slightly bent. Both the man and woman place their hands to the sides of their heads. Be sure not to interlace your fingers behind the head—this may cause a strain to your neck muscles. Working together, alternate your feet position and bring the opposite elbow to the bent knee. Do this at a slower pace. Do 10–15 reps for 3 sets.

COMBONATION #34
PUSH DOWNS

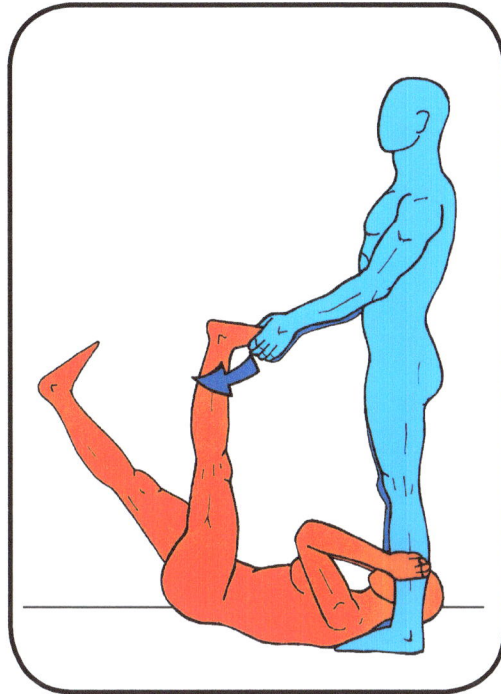

Figure 4-29

Muscles Worked:

Man and Woman: Rectus abdominis
and iliopsoas, *internal obliques

The man stands upright, with his feet slightly less than shoulder-width apart. The woman lies in a supine position, placing her head between the man's feet, grabbing his ankles and elevating her legs until they are perpendicular to the mat. The man grabs the woman's feet and pushes them away using moderate force. The woman attempts to prevent her feet from touching the floor then raises her legs again to her partner, back at the starting position.

*The obliques can be worked as well by pushing the legs to the sides. This is a more advanced abdominal exercise, so start moderately then increase when comfortable. Do 5–10 reps in each direction

CHAPTER FIVE
COOLDOWN AND POST PLAY

To this point we have covered all the major components of an exercise program: warm-up, stretch, and exercise. We have also discussed the correlation and benefits of foreplay and sex in relation to warm-up and exercise, respectively. Now we must address the final component, one that is often overlooked and underappreciated, this is the **Cooldown** period.

The purpose of the cooldown period is to slowly decrease the heart rate and metabolism, which have been elevated during physical activity. A low-level aerobic exercise, similar to that of the physical activity, is recommended. Jogging, walking, and cycling are some good examples. The cooldown period helps prevent sudden pooling of blood in the veins and facilitates adequate circulation to the skeletal muscles, heart, and the brain. There are several risks associated with sudden cessation of exercise. Some examples are: muscle soreness, improper cardiac function due to high concentrations of adrenaline in the blood, and fainting and dizziness. Cooldown should also be followed by five to ten minutes of stretching to avoid Delayed-Onset Muscle Soreness (DOMS).

We shall now look at a relatively new term that correlates with the cooldown period but has not been defined by Webster. Therefore the definition will reflect my philosophical views. **Post Play** is the period and actions that follow the act of intimacy. In chapter one, I touched on the subject briefly when defining the refractory period. In this chapter, we will further explore the benefits and possibilities of the post play period.

Just as the cooldown is an integral part of the exercise program, post play in relation to sex is every bit as important for several reasons: 1) it slowly brings the heart rate and metabolism back down to its normal level, 2) it prolongs the euphoric feeling or state that follows orgasm through continued body contact, and 3) it offers couples an opportunity to converse with their guards down.

Just as foreplay is an issue of great concern for women, post play is no less important. The creative mind can use this time wisely to appease their mate by doing the small things. Personally, I like this time because my wife and I can talk about different topics as we lie there embracing one another or while we take a soothing hot shower together..

I do not look at the act of intimacy as intercourse alone. I view it as an art form—as it was described to me many years ago. My pleasure does not begin and end with the physical release—it is in pleasing my spouse through all three stages of the act, knowing she will please me in return. Here are some tips for those who would like to add variety.

TIPS

1. After you and your partner have reached fulfillment, the man and or the woman can get a washcloth and wash his or her partner up. He or she will be very grateful for this act of kindness.

2. Continue to remain in contact with your partner by either placing a leg across their leg or a hand that gently caresses the skin. This will assure them that you are still connected emotionally and that it was about more than your own pleasure.

3. Have an intimate conversation discussing the experience, work, the family, or future plans.

4. Take a nice hot bath or shower with your partner so you can continue the conversation as well as take turns washing each other up.

5. After exiting the shower, dry one another off and apply body lotion on each other's skin to help keep it soft and to replace moisture that was lost. This would be the perfect time to rub the body down and further relax the muscles and the mind.

6. If the experience was so taxing that you do not have the energy to do all these other things right away, simply embrace one another and fall asleep in each other's arms.

These are but a few tips that I have found to be very beneficial and pleasurable from my experience. To all the readers, please take heed of these things I say, be attentive to your mate, creative with your mind, and utilize this time wisely.

CHAPTER SIX
MASSAGE

When Combocising was first conceived, my idea consisted only of combining calisthenics exercise and intimacy, but as I furthered my education in the area of massage, I saw the importance of adding this component to the program. Massage is an excellent adjunct therapy for several reasons: 1) It facilitates muscle growth and speedy muscle recovery, 2) relieves tension and stress, 3) improves blood circulation, and 4) it is an excellent means of communicating sensual thoughts.

Studies have shown the many benefits of this ancient art form, which is depicted in the murals of the pyramids in Egypt. Western civilization is beginning to understand and accept this art form slowly, but we have considerable ground to cover. This was evident by the results of a survey I conducted while in the Start Your Own Business Class. I interviewed sixty-five men and women, ranging in ages from eighteen to fifty-plus, and of varying educational and occupational background. In relation to massage, when they were asked, "Does your significant other offer to massage you?" The responses were as follows:

- 9% regularly

- 49% sometimes

- 18% rarely

- 15% never

- **9**% did not respond

Out of sixty-five people, only six individuals received massages from their partner on a regular basis. This was pretty astonishing, considering that the overwhelming majority of people wanted to receive massage an average of two times per month. There are many factors that prevent people from receiving professional therapeutic massage; the most noted reasons are affordability and lack of knowledge of the benefits.

With affordability being one of the top inhibitors, this is all the more reason why couples should learn to administer a healing touch as well as a sensual one. We are living in uncertain times, where there is the threat of war continually on the horizon, parents killing kids, and kids killing their parents. A time where we have created a standard of living that has turned us into economic slaves, forcing both parents into the workforce, leaving our kids to be raised by society and Hollywood.

Every day tension is high; I can feel it as I work on my clients, trying to bring them some relief from their day to day struggles. Besides muscle aches, this type of muscle tension can cause headaches and illness. Yes, I said illness—this is because stress inhibits the body's immune system from fighting sickness and disease. Excessive stress can manifest as cardiovascular disorders, including hypertension; digestive difficulties such as heartburn, ulcers, and bowl syndrome; respiratory illness, sleep disorders, and bacterial and viral illness, to name a few.

When these disorders or illnesses arise, the first thing most of us have a tendency to do is to call up Dr. Frankenstein for help, only to be poked and prodded like lab rats or guinea pigs and given mind- and body-altering drugs. For example, an article written in the local newspaper (*The Morning Call*) reported that many Americans might be poisoning their livers by unwittingly taking toxic doses of acetaminophen, also known as the Tylenol brand. This is but one drug that has raised concerns, but there are hundreds, even thousands, that are on the market, causing harm, even death, to the unsuspecting.

What most people need to realize is that we have more control over our own well-being than they (meaning the doctors and pharmaceutical companies) would like us to know. A sensible diet, plenty of water and rest, and a fitness and weight training program incorporated in your daily lives can and should be used as preventive maintenance. These are some of the components that contribute to optimal heath and fitness, but massage is perhaps the most overlooked and underappreciated of them all. So don't wait for your significant other to be in pain before asking if you can rub their back. Take it upon yourself to relieve some of the day-to-day stress with a soothing touch.

I will now give you some of the basic do's and don'ts of massage, but before you and your partner begin to administer full-body massages to each other, I recommend that you do one of three things: 1) Read a book, 2) Watch a video tape, or 3) Take a class on massage therapy.

Massage is a beautiful and useful art form, but it can be harmful if applied incorrectly. There are several things that a person administering massage must be made aware of:

1) stay in constant contact with your partner, continually asking about the pressure— whether it's too light or too great.

2) Always apply the stroke going in the direction of the heart.

3) Stay away from endangerment zones such as arteries, lymph node glands, major nerve plexuses.

4) Avoid massaging areas with broken skin.

5) Inquire as to the types of medications the person may be on, if any.

6) Avoid massage swollen or inflamed areas immediately after injury.

7) Do not massage an individual who is ill.

This chapter is not intended to train individuals in massage therapy, only to suggest the benefits and importance thereof. The following illustrations, figures 4-61 through 4-63 on pages 69 through 71, demonstrate several intimate positions that incorporate calisthenics and massage. Refer to chapter 1, page 18, figure 1-2 for cranial massage and chapter 4, page 37, figure 4-6 for a variation of male back massage. Since time does not always appear to be on our side, these combonations show how two birds can be killed with one stone, as the old cliché goes.

COMBONATION #35
BACK MASSAGE

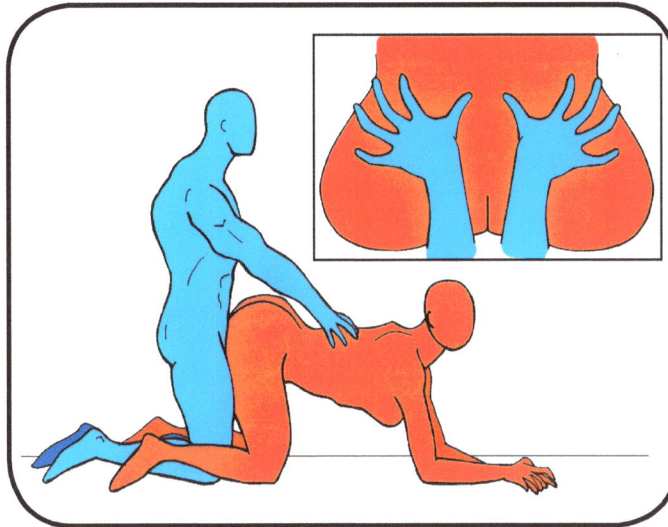

Figure 6-1

Muscles Worked: Entire back and gluteal muscles

The woman assumes the "doggy style" position—on her hands and knees. The man kneels down and positions himself to enter her from behind. He then begins to gently massage the woman's upper, middle, and lower back. Do not apply too much pressure while massaging. The gluteal muscles (buttocks) can also be massaged. Take this time to soothe and relax her troubled areas and channel positive energy into her. There are no time limits for this action.

COMBONATION #36
MASSAGE, SQUATS, AND ROLL UPS

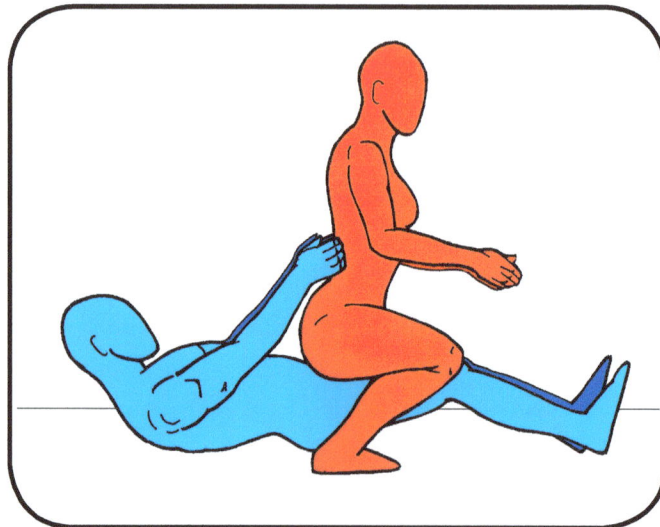

Figure 6-2

Muscles Massaged:

Middle and lower back

Muscles Worked:

Man: Upper and middle rectus abdominis

Woman: Quadraceps femoris group and gluteus maximus

The man lies in a supine position, with his legs slightly bent. Facing away from the man, the woman straddles him, lowers herself to the squat position, and inserts his penis into her vagina. She begins by pushing up using her legs, then lowering herself back to the starting position and repeating this action 10–12 times for 3 sets. The woman may also increase the intensity and pleasure by gyrating in either the up or down position.

The man rises up, performing partial sit-ups while massaging the woman's middle and lower back. The man should try to hold each sit-up for 2–3 seconds before lowering himself back to the mat. Do this for 10–15 reps for 3 sets.

COMBONATION #37
MASSAGE AND LATERAL TWIST
OR SIDE-LYING LATERAL CRUNCHES

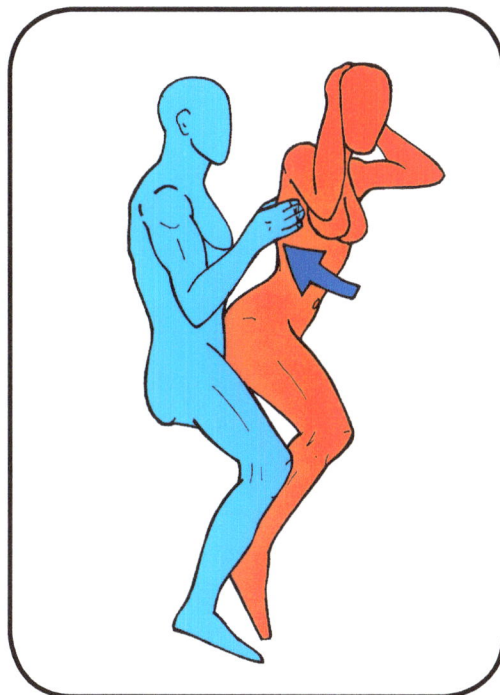

Figure 6-3

Muscles Massaged:
Upper and middle and lower back
Muscle Worked: External and internal obliques

Both the man and woman lie on their sides, with the woman in front of the man. The man enters from behind then begins to massage the woman's upper, middle, and lower back. The woman places her hands to the sides of her head and begins to perform lateral twists by lifting her torso off the mat, bringing the elbow closest to the floor to the opposite knee, then lowering herself back down to the mat. After completing the predetermined number of reps, the man and woman come close together as the man wraps his arms around the woman and rolls to the other side and repeats the exercise. Do 10–15 reps for 3 sets on each side.

CHAPTER SEVEN
NUTRITION AND DIETING

Nutrition and dieting are very subjective because every individual is different and has different needs. For example, a person trying to lose or maintain a certain weight has different nutritional and dietary needs than a person training for a 10K marathon.

The market is flooded with hundreds of diets. Ones that work for some don't work for others, and many just don't work at all. In chapter 2 on page 19, I stated that everything you eat is a part of your diet, so rather than to starve yourself, find out what the body needs nutritionally and what you must do to get it.

Before we go any further, though, perhaps we should define what nutrients are. Nutrients are life-sustaining substances found in food. Together they work to supply the body with energy and structural materials and to regulate growth, maintenance, and repair of the body tissue. The six major classes of nutrients are **Proteins, Carbohydrates, Fats, Vitamins, Minerals, and Water.** Table 7-1 below lists the six classes of nutrients and their major functions.

Table 7-1 Six Classes of Nutrients

Nutrient	Function
Protein	- builds & repairs body tissue - major component of enzymes, harmones & antibodies
Carbohydrate	- provides a major source of fuel to the body - provides dietary fibers
Lipids	- chief storage form of energy in the body - insulate and protect vital organs - provide fat-soluble vitamins
Vitamins	- help promote & regulate various chemical reactions & bodily processes - Do not yeild energy themselves, but participate in releasing energy from food
Minerals	- Enable enzymes to function - a component of harmones - a part of bone & nerve impulses
Water	- enables chemical reactions to occur - about 60% of the body is composed of water - essential for life as we connot store it, nor conserve it

The amounts needed from each class vary widely, but it is important that the body receives enough in order to achieve optimal health and maintain an active lifestyle. The body is an incredible work of art and can produce certain nutrients from others. For instance, the body can convert some amino acids into carbohydrates and can produce some vitamins from amino acids. However, there are certain compounds called essential amino acids that the body cannot manufacture for itself. These essential amino acids are just that—essential to the maximal production of the body's day-to-day activities.

There are said to be about forty essential nutrients that we should be concerned with. Do not let this number alarm you, however. With proper dietary planning, you can take in all of the necessary nutrients needed to maintain optimal health.

Table 7-2 on page 74 is the My Pyramid, Steps To A Healthier You food guideline. These guidelines were developed by the United States Department of Agriculture Center for Policy and Promotion in April of 2005, replacing the food pyramid that was introduced in 1992. The My Pyramid system lists a variety of food choices chosen from the five food groups. This chart, in combination with table 7-3 on page 75 lays out the dietary guidelines and gives you the major contributors from each food group.

My Pyramid simplifies the dietary guidelines by turning it into real food choices. Be sure to eat at least the lowest number of servings from the five major food groups listed. This will give you the vitamins, minerals, carbohydrates, and proteins needed, but try to pick the lowest-fat choices from the food groups.

There are several other things to consider when planning your diet:

1) Balance your diet with physical activity to control and improve your weight.
2) A diet should be low in total fat, saturated fat, and cholesterol.
3) A diet should consist of plenty of vegetables, fruits, and grain products.
4) A diet should be moderate in sugar.
5) A diet should be moderate in salt and sodium.
6) If you are trying to lose weight avoid the three whites: flour, sugar, and salt.

For more information, go to (http://www.mypyramid.gov).

Table 7-2 My Pyramid

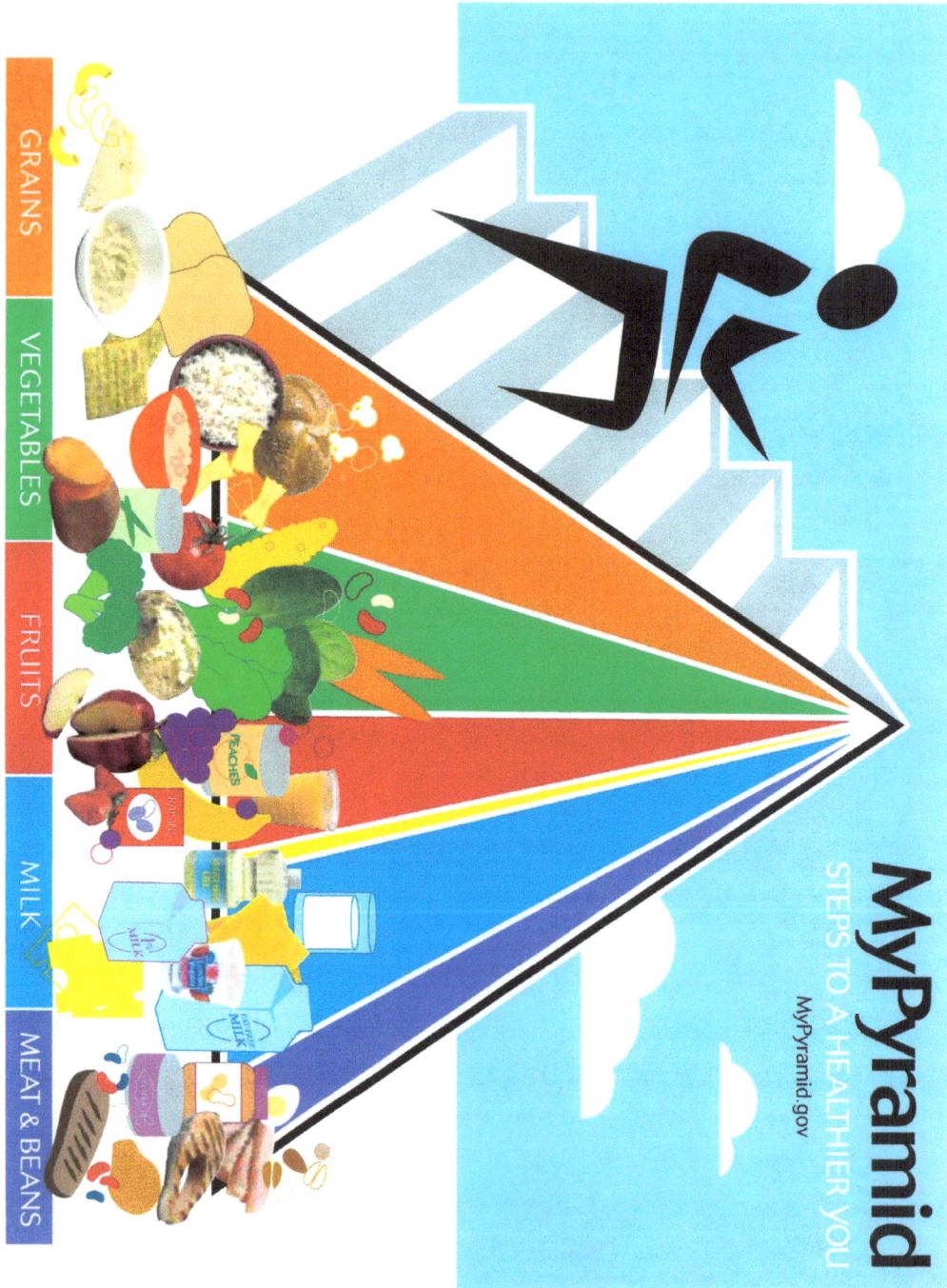

MyPyramid
STEPS TO A HEALTHIER YOU
MyPyramid.gov

GRAINS   VEGETABLES   FRUITS   MILK   MEAT & BEANS

Table 7-3 My Pyramid Summary

Food Group	Servings	Major Contributions	Food & Sering Size
Milk, Yogurt, Cheese	2-3 adult; 3-4 children, teens, pregnant or lactating	Calcium Carbohydrate Ribflavin, Protein Zinc, Potassium	1 cup of milk 1 ½ ounce of cheese 1 cup yogurt 2 cups cottage cheese 1 cup pudding
Meat, Poultry, Fish, Dry Bean, Eggs & Nuts	2-3	Protein, Niacin, Iron, Vitamin B6, Zinc, Thiamin, Vitamin B12	2-3 ounces of meat, poultry or fish; 1 ½ cups beans 2 Tbsp. peanut butter 2 eggs, ½ -1 cup nuts
Fruits	2-4	Carbohydrate Vitamin C, Fiber	¼ cup dried fruit ½ cup cooked fruit ¾ cup juice 1 whole piece of fruit
Vegetables	3-5	Carbohydrate, Vitamin A, Vitamin C, Folate Magnesium Dietary Fiber	½ cup raw or cooked 1 cup leafy greens ½ cup vegetable juice
Bread, Cereals Rice & Pasta	6-11	Carbohydrate Thiamin, Iron Niacin, Folate Magnesium Dietary Fiber	1 slice of bread 1 ounce of cereal ½ - ¾ cup cooked cereal, pasta or rice
Fats, Oils & Sweets	Foods from this group should not replace any from the other groups. Amounts consumed should be determined by individual energy needs.		

As with everything, variety is important, as is moderation. The food guide chart does not dictate the food that you can eat. It was devised so that you could make sound decisions on what you should eat. There are substitute foods in every food group, which gives the individual plenty of choices to pick from. Table 7-2 on page 74 gives you the food groups, servings, major contributors, and food servings and sizes while tables 7-4 and 7-5 on pages 77 through 79 list the vitamins and minerals, USRDA, best sources, and functions.

Many people take the route of using dietary supplements; I personally have several views on this issue: 1) If your schedule is so hectic that you cannot put in place a system that will allow you to eat a balanced diet, then I can see the necessity in taking supplements. 2) If you are willing to make the necessary changes in your lifestyle that can afford you a better meal, a more complete meal, then supplements are unnecessary. 3) The FDA (Food and Drug Administration) does not regulate supplements. The Dietary Supplement Health and Education Act of 1994 prevents the FDA from recalling any substance unless it has been proven to pose a danger.

This statement in and of itself should raise concern for the estimated two million men and one million women who use ephedrine. Ephedrine is marketed as a weight-loss aid and energy booster. Recent reports have linked this supplement to major health conditions, including heart attacks. This again is but one of many products on the market that may cause serious harm to the unsuspecting consumer. So before you begin taking any supplements, do the research, and maybe you'll find what your looking for in a natural form.

Don't get me wrong, I understand chaotic schedules and time constraints—I am a very busy man myself—but at the same time, I realize that if I do not take proper care of myself now, I will inherit health problems later in life. Understand that the body works on a very acute chemical balance. If something is added that does not correspond with the body's natural order of operation, you will suffer from what are commonly known as side effects.

These are often associated with prescription drugs, but studies are now finding that supplements and over the counter drugs are potentially dangerous due to the accumulative effect. I theorize that many of the people taking supplements to enhance their appearance or performance will develop illnesses associated with the heart, kidneys, and the liver in the next ten to twenty years.

Table 7-4 Vitamin Chart

Vitamin	U.S. RDA	Best Sources	Functions
A (carotene)	5,000 IU/day	Yellow or orange fruits and vegetables, green leafy vegetables, fortified oatmeal, liver, dairy products	Formation and maintenance of skin, hair and mucous membranes; Helps you see in dim light; bone and tooth growth
B 1 (thiamine)	1.5 mg/day	Fortified cereals and Oatmeal's, meats, rice and Pasta, whole grains, liver	Helps body release energy from carbohydrates during Metabolism; growth and muscle tone
B 2 (riboflavin)	1.7 mg/day	Whole grains, green leafy Vegetables, organ meats, Milk and eggs	Helps body release energy protein, fat & carbohydrates during metabolism
B 6 (pyridoxine)	2mg/day	Fish, poultry, lean meats, Bananas, prunes, dried Beans, whole grains, Avocados	Helps build body tissue and aids in metabolism of protein
B 12 (cobalamin)	6 mcg/day	Meats, milk products, seafood	Aids cell development, Functioning of the nervous System & the metabolism of protein and fat
Biotin	.3 mg/day	Cereal /grain products yeast, legumes, liver	Involved in metabolism of protein, fats & carbohydrates
Folate (folacin, folic acid)	.4 mg/day	Green leafy vegetables, organ meats, dried peas, beans and lentils	Aids in genetic material development and involved in red blood cell production
Niacin	20 mg/day	Meat, poultry, fish, cereals Peanuts, potatoes, dairy products, eggs	involved in carbohydrate, protein and fat metabolism
Pantothenic acid	10 mg/day	Lean meats, whole grains legumes, vegetables, fruit	Helps release energy from fats and carbohydrates
C (absorbic acid)	60 mg/day	Citrus fruits, berries & vegetables – especially peppers	Essential for structure of bones, muscle, cartilage, & blood vessels; maintains capillaries and gums & gums & aids in absorption of iron

Table 7-4 Vitamin Chart (Contd.)

Vitamin	U.S. RDA	Best Sources	Functions
D	400 IU/day	Fortified milk, sunlight, fish, eggs, butter, fortified margarine	Aids in bone and tooth formation; helps maintain heart action & nervous system
E	30 IU/day	Fortified and multi-grain Cereals, nuts, wheat germ vegetable oils, green leafy vegetable	Protects blood cells, body tissue & essential fatty acids from harmful destruction in body
K	**	Green leafy vegetables, fruit, dairy	Essential for blood clothing functions

Table 7-5 Mineral Chart

Vitamin	U.S. RDA	Best Sources	Functions
Calcium	1000 mg/day	Milk & milk products	Strong bones, teeth, muscles tissue; regulates heartbeat, muscle action & nerve function; blood clotting
Chromium	no RDA	corn oil, clams grain cereals	Glucose metabolism (energy); increases effectiveness of insulin
Copper	2 mg/day	Oysters, nuts, organ meats, legumes	Formation of red blood cells, bones growth & health; works with vitamin C to form elastin
Iodine	150 mcg/day	Seafood, iodized salt	Component of hormone thyroxin, which controls metabolism
Iron	18 mg/day	Meats & organ meats, legumes	Hemoglobin formation; improves blood quality; increases resistance to stress & disease
Magnesium	no RDA	Nuts, vegetables whole grains	Acid/ alkaline balance; important in metabolism of carbohydrates, minerals & sugars

Table 7-5 Mineral Chart (Contd.)

Vitamin	U.S. RDA	Best Sources	Functions
Manganese	no RDA	Nuts, grains, vegetables, fruit	Enzyme activation; carbohydrate & fat production; sex hormone production; skeletal development
Phosphorus	1000 mg/day	Fish, meat, eggs poultry, grains	Bone development; important in protein, fat & carbohydrate utilization
Potassium	no RDA	Lean meat, fruit, vegetables	Fluid balance; controls activity of heart muscle, nervous system, kidneys
Selenium	50-200 mcg/day	Seafood, organ meats, grains, lean meats	Protects body tissues against oxidative damage from radiation, pollution & normal metabolic processing
Zinc	15 mg/day	Lean meats, egg liver, seafood, whole grains	Involved in digestion & metabolism, important in development of reproductive system, aids in healing

Please do not be fooled by companies that tell you that their products are all–natural. This is often a marketing and advertisement trick. When the body or nature creates a substance, then and only then is it natural, but if it is synthesized in a laboratory and compressed into pill form with chemical additives, then there is little that is natural about that product. A proper diet combined with a fitness/weight training program will help you maintain your weight and health without the use of supplements.

Continued education will bring you a better understanding of what the body needs to remain healthy and help you avoid all of the charlatans and gimmicks they have to offer. For many, this will seem like an impossible task, but the first step in achieving success is being critical of yourself. The second step is wanting to make change. The third step is accepting change. Once you get started, it will become routine and get easier with each day. Though there will be those times when you just don't feel up to it, stay disciplined and fight through it.

ADDITIONAL WEIGHT LOSS AND MAINTENANCE TIPS

1. Face the reality. There is no quick fix to the weight loss problem. It takes discipline and hard work.

2. Increasing muscle mass speeds up your metabolism. Calories are units of energy that are abundant in fat and are broken down to sustain the required levels of energy.

3. Look in the mirror and picture yourself the way you want to look in several weeks.

4. Keep your eye on the prize.

5. Plan your dinner so that there are 2–3 hours of digestion before bedtime.

6. Cut out late-night snacks.

7. Eat foods low in saturated fat.

8. Eat several smaller portions of food throughout the day rather than three square meals.

9. Take a picture before you begin a fitness/weight training program. This, along with baseline weight and body fat percentages, will allow you to measure your gains.

10. Eat foods high in fiber.

11. Eat healthy snacks such as fruits and vegetables instead of highly processed junk.

12. Continue to educate yourself about the body's functions and needs.

13. Stay busy. An idle mind has plenty of time to think about snacks and goodies.

14. Love yourself for who you are. It is important for you to realize God makes no mistakes.

15. Change because of your own needs and desires, not those of society.

CHAPTER EIGHT
EXERCISE AND RELATIONSHIPS

To this point, we have discussed the correlation between the components of exercise, fitness, and sex. Now let us begin to examine exercise and the relationship as a whole.

Exercise when performed with a partner is centered on teamwork and founded on unity and communication. **Teamwork** is defined as joint action by a group of people in which individual interest is subordinated to group unity and efficiency. **Unity** is defined as something complete in itself, the quality of being one in spirit. **Communication** is the ability to express ideas verbally or in written form. Marriages and relationships follow the same principles, with the written or unwritten assumption that the parties involved will have a vested interest in the other's welfare.

People form bonds based on many different things and on many different levels. Unfortunately, sometimes interests change over the years, and people more often than not tend to drift apart from one another. Exercise and fitness are great forums on which to bond because one thing that remains a constant in our everyday lives is the issue of health. Whether you choose Combocising, running, walking, cycling, or aerobics, the time spent together with your significant other will be of great benefit. This is especially true since we all want to be healthy and stay healthy even though most of us do not do what is necessary to maintain good health. This can sometimes be blamed on a lack of knowledge and other times complacency or laziness, but many times it is a lack of support. One of the many definitions of **support** is to give courage, faith, or confidence; to help or comfort.

As a personal trainer and consultant, I often have to ask questions pertaining to the client's support system (family and friends). Surprisingly, most people don't have the support necessary from family and friends to keep them motivated. Consequently they hit bumps in the road and become discouraged and eventually discontinue their program. This however should not be the case, especially in marriage, where we pledge to one another vows to stay together through thick and through thin, through sickness and through health, until death do you us part. It means that we should always be there for one another until the end of our days. This statement should not be taken lightly. For the Bible says that "tomorrow is promised to no man," therefore no man knows when his day will come. You see, time is a precious gift given to us, and once time passes, you can never get it back.

I have seen and heard of many cases where family members, friends, and people in general waited until they were diagnosed with a terminal illness before they began to realize how precious and short life really is. In the motion picture *Things to Do in Denver When You're Dead*, starring Andy Garcia, one of the characters described life as going by faster than summer vacation. That was probably the most profound statement in the whole movie, and it has been etched in my mind for years. There is validity to this statement.

Think back to when you were in elementary, junior, or high school—how fast those summer days flew by. Now look at you: most of you reading this book are in your twenties, thirties, forties, even fifties, wondering where the time went. If we are fortunate enough to live until we are seventy years old, this will roughly equate to 613,608 hours. If we live accordingly and break the day down into thirds, using eight hours for work, eight hours for leisure time, and 8 hours for rest, we actually have only 204,331.5 hours of conscious time to divide amongst our choirs, family, and friends. As you can clearly see, in the whole scheme of things, this is very little time. So regardless of how you choose to do it, make sure you spend as much time as possible with the one or ones you love.

NOTES

Note 1): Not all combonations are for every individual. Choose the exercise positions that best meet your needs, desires, and fitness level.

Note 2): If you suffer from high blood pressure, coronary disease, back injury, or any other physically disabling or limiting condition; contact a physician before beginning an exercise program.

Note 3): Men forty years and older and women fifty years and older should see a doctor and get a physical release and recommendation.

Note 4): When attempting to lose weight, a person should lose no more than two or three pounds a week. For example, if your goal is to lose twenty pounds, allow yourself ten weeks to reach your goal.

Note 5): The program can be performed with or without clothing on. However, greater arousal and anticipation can be achieved when performed with just enough clothing to excite your imagination.

Note 6): To fully maximize the workout program, allow the exercises to lead you into the act of intimacy.

Note 7): If you are new to fitness or just getting back into it, start off slow and gradually increase the number of repetitions and sets.

Note 8): Do not overwork the muscles. This could cause muscle soreness, irritability, loss of sleep, and possible muscle injury.

SAMPLE WORKOUT PROGRAM I

Monday

Warm-up: dance and stretch, 15–20 min.
Figures: 3-1 pg. 24, 3-2 pg. 25, 3-3 pg. 26, 3-4 pg. 27

Chest
Figures: 4-1 pg. 32, 4-2 pg. 33, 4-3 pg. 34, 4-9 pg. 40

Triceps
Figures: 4-14 pg. 45, 4-15 pg. 46, 4-16 pg. 47, 4-17 pg. 48

Wednesday
Warm-up: dance and stretch, 15–20 min.
Figures: 3-1 pg. 24, 3-2 pg. 25, 3-3 pg. 26, 3-4 pg. 27

Back
Figures: 4-10 pg. 41, 4-11 pg. 42, 4-12 pg. 43, 4-13 pg. 44

Biceps
Figures: 4-14 pg. 45, 4-15 pg. 46

Friday
Warm-up: dance and stretch, 15–20 min.
Figures: 3-1 pg. 24, 3-2 pg. 25, 3-3 pg. 26, 3-4 pg. 27

Shoulders
Figures: 4-18 pg. 50, 4-19 pg. 51

Legs
Figures: 4-20 pg. 53, 4-21 pg. 54, 4-22 pg. 55, 4-24 pg. 57, 4-25 pg. 58, 4-26 pg. 59
Sample Workout Program 2

84 | COMBOCISING

FULL BODY WORKOUT

Tuesday

Warm-up: dance and stretch, 15–20 min.

 Figures: 3-1 pg. 24, 3-2 pg. 25, 3-3 pg. 26, 3-4 pg. 27

Chest

Figures: 4-1 pg. 32, 4-3 pg. 34

Shoulders

Figures: 4-18 pg. 50, 4-19 pg. 51

Back

Figures: 4-10 pg. 41, 4-13 pg. 44

Arms

Figures: 4-14 pg. 45, 4-15 pg. 46 (biceps)

Figures: 4-16 pg. 47, 4-17 pg. 48 (triceps)

Legs

Figures: 4-21 pg. 54, 4-24 pg. 57, 4-26 pg. 59

Friday

Warm-up: dance and stretch, 15–20 min.

 Figures: 3-1 pg. 24, 3-2 pg. 25, 3-3 pg. 26, 3-4 pg. 27

Chest

Figures: 4-1 pg. 32, 4-3 pg. 34

Shoulders

Figures: 4-18 pg. 50, 4-19 pg. 51

Back
Figures: 4-10 pg. 41, 4-13 pg. 44

Arms
Figures: 4-14 pg. 45, 4-15 pg. 46 (biceps)
Figures: 4-16 pg. 47, 4-17 pg. 48 (triceps)

Legs
Figures: 4-21 pg. 54, 4-24 pg. 57, 4-26 pg. 59

Aditional Chest Excercises
Figures: 4-4 pg. 35, 4-5 pg.36, 4-6 pg. 37, 4-7 pg. 38, 4-8 pg. 39

Aditional Core Excercises
Figures: 1-2 pg. 18, 4-27 pg.61, 4-28 pg. 62, 4-29 pg. 63

Massage
Figures: 6-1 pg. 69, 6-2 pg. 70, 6-3 pg. 71

TRAINING LOG

Name		Age		Sex		Fitness hx.			
Warm-up (5-10 min.) Stretching (hold 10 sec.) Strengthening Cardiovascular (20 min.+) Cool down									
Exercise name	Date								
	Reps.								
	Sets.								
	Reps.								
	Sets.								
	Reps.								
	Sets.								
	Reps.								
	Sets.								
	Reps.								
	Sets.								
	Reps.								
	Sets.								
	Reps.								
	Sets.								
	Reps.								
	Sets.								
	Reps.								
	Sets.								
	Reps.								
	Sets.								
	Reps.								
	Sets.								
	Reps.								
	Sets.								
	Reps.								
	Sets.								

TRAINING LOG

Name	Age		Sex			Fitness hx.		
Warm-up (5-10 min.) Stretching (hold 10 sec.) Strengthening Cardiovascular (20 min.+) Cool down								
Exercise name	Date							
	Reps.							
	Sets.							
	Reps.							
	Sets.							
	Reps.							
	Sets.							
	Reps.							
	Sets.							
	Reps.							
	Sets.							
	Reps.							
	Sets.							
	Reps.							
	Sets.							
	Reps.							
	Sets.							
	Reps.							
	Sets.							
	Reps.							
	Sets.							
	Reps.							
	Sets.							
	Reps.							
	Sets.							
	Reps.							
	Sets.							
	Reps.							
	Sets.							

TRAINING LOG

Name		Age		Sex		Fitness hx.			
Warm-up (5-10 min.) Stretching (hold 10 sec.) Strengthening Cardiovascular (20 min.+) Cool down									
Exercise name	Date								
	Reps.								
	Sets.								
	Reps.								
	Sets.								
	Reps.								
	Sets.								
	Reps.								
	Sets.								
	Reps.								
	Sets.								
	Reps.								
	Sets.								
	Reps.								
	Sets.								
	Reps.								
	Sets.								
	Reps.								
	Scts.								
	Reps.								
	Sets.								
	Reps.								
	Sets.								
	Reps.								
	Sets.								
	Reps.								
	Sets.								
	Reps.								
	Sets.								

TRAINING LOG

Name	Age	Sex	Fitness hx.
Warm-up (5-10 min.) Stretching (hold 10 sec.) Strengthening Cardiovascular (20 min.+) Cool down			

Exercise name	Date								
	Reps.								
	Sets.								
	Reps.								
	Sets.								
	Reps.								
	Sets.								
	Reps.								
	Sets.								
	Reps.								
	Sets.								
	Reps.								
	Sets.								
	Reps.								
	Sets.								
	Reps.								
	Sets.								
	Reps.								
	Sets.								
	Reps.								
	Sets.								
	Reps.								
	Sets.								
	Reps.								
	Sets.								
	Reps.								
	Sets.								
	Reps.								
	Sets.								

TRAINING LOG

Name		Age		Sex		Fitness hx.		
Warm-up (5-10 min.) Stretching (hold 10 sec.) Strengthening Cardiovascular (20 min.+) Cool down								
Exercise name	Date							
	Reps.							
	Sets.							
	Reps.							
	Sets.							
	Reps.							
	Sets.							
	Reps.							
	Sets.							
	Reps.							
	Sets.							
	Reps.							
	Sets.							
	Reps.							
	Sets.							
	Reps.							
	Sets.							
	Reps.							
	Sets.							
	Reps.							
	Sets.							
	Reps.							
	Sets.							
	Reps.							
	Sets.							
	Reps.							
	Sets.							

TRAINING LOG

Name	Age		Sex			Fitness hx.		
Warm-up (5-10 min.) Stretching (hold 10 sec.) Strengthening Cardiovascular (20 min.+) Cool down								
Exercise name	Date							
	Reps.							
	Sets.							
	Reps.							
	Sets.							
	Reps.							
	Sets.							
	Reps.							
	Sets.							
	Reps.							
	Sets.							
	Reps.							
	Sets.							
	Reps.							
	Sets.							
	Reps.							
	Sets.							
	Reps.							
	Sets.							
	Reps.							
	Sets.							
	Reps.							
	Sets.							
	Reps.							
	Sets.							
	Reps.							
	Sets.							
	Reps.							
	Sets.							

TRAINING LOG

Name		Age		Sex		Fitness hx.		
Warm-up (5-10 min.) Stretching (hold 10 sec.) Strengthening Cardiovascular (20 min.+) Cool down								
Exercise name	Date							
	Reps.							
	Sets.							
	Reps.							
	Sets.							
	Reps.							
	Sets.							
	Reps.							
	Sets.							
	Reps.							
	Sets.							
	Reps.							
	Sets.							
	Reps.							
	Sets.							
	Reps.							
	Sets.							
	Reps.							
	Sets.							
	Reps.							
	Sets.							
	Reps.							
	Sets.							
	Reps.							
	Sets.							
	Reps.							
	Sets.							
	Reps.							
	Sets.							
	Reps.							
	Sets.							

TRAINING LOG

Name	Age		Sex		Fitness hx.		
Warm-up (5-10 min.) Stretching (hold 10 sec.) Strengthening Cardiovascular (20 min.+) Cool down							
Exercise name	Date						
	Reps.						
	Sets.						
	Reps.						
	Sets.						
	Reps.						
	Sets.						
	Reps.						
	Sets.						
	Reps.						
	Sets.						
	Reps.						
	Sets.						
	Reps.						
	Sets.						
	Reps.						
	Sets.						
	Reps.						
	Sets.						
	Reps.						
	Sets.						
	Reps.						
	Sets.						
	Reps.						
	Sets.						
	Reps.						
	Sets.						
	Reps.						
	Sets.						

REFERENCE PAGE

- Applegate, E. 2000. The anatomy and physiology learning system (2nd ed.). Philadelphia: W.B. Saunders Company.

- Bridges, A. (2006, Dec.). FDA seeks stricter warnings on pain relievers. The Morning Call, pp. A9. (Associated Press).

- Chia, M. and D. Abrams. 1996. The multi-orgasmic man: How any man can experience multiple orgasms and dramatically enhance his sexual relationship. New York: Harper Collins.

- Chia, M. and R. C. Abrams. 2005. The multi-orgasmic woman: Discover your full desire, pleasure, and vitality.United States: Rodale Inc.

- Cotton, R. T., and C. J. Ekeroth, eds. 1996. Lifestyle and weight management: Consultant manual. San Diego: American Council on Exercise.

- Cotton, R. T., and C. J. Ekeroth, eds. 1996, 1997. Personal trainer manual: The resource for fitness professionals. San Diego

- Chapman, G. D. 1995. The five love languages: How to express heartfelt commitment to your mate. Chicago: Northfield.

- Fleder, G., director. 1995. Things to do in Denver when you're dead [Motion picture]. United States: Miramax.

- Fritz S. 2000. Mosby's fundamentals of therapeutic massage (2nd ed.). St. Louis

- Gerard, J. 2001. Can exercise improve your sex life? *Fitness Matters, Volume 7*, 8-10.

- Guralnik, D.B. 1997. Webster's New World Dictionary (3rd ed.) College. New York: Macmillan.

- O'Neill H. 1997, November. Surprising health benefits of sex. *Men's Health*, 29- 33, 36.

- Rubin, J. P. 2002. Sports based relationships: The ties that bind. *Fitness Matters, Volume 8,* 12-13.

- Sieg, K. W. , S. P. Adams. 1996. Illustrated essentials of musculoskeletal anatomy (3rd ed.). Gainesville: Megabooks Inc.

- U.S. Department of Agriculture. Food and Drug Administration. 1994. The Dietary Supplement Health and Education Act. Retrieved January 2, 2002, from **http:// www.usda.gov**

- Wuh, H. C.K. and M. Fox. 2002. Sexual fitness: 7 essential elements to optimizing your sensuality, satisfaction, and well-being. New York: Penguin Group Inc.

www.ingramcontent.com/pod-product-compliance
Lightning Source LLC
Chambersburg PA
CBHW060802270326
41926CB00002B/59